The Effective Management of Benign Prostatic Disease and Lower Urinary Tract Symptoms

The Effective Management of Benign Prostatic Disease and Lower Urinary Tract Symptoms

Edited by

Tom McNicholas MB BS FRCS FEBU
Consultant Urological Surgeon, Lister Hospital, Stevenage

Michael Kirby MB BS MRCP
*General Practitioner, and Director of HertNet, The Hertfordshire
Primary Care Research Network, University of Hertfordshire, Hatfield*

Andrew Miles MSc MPhil PhD
*UeL Professor of Health Services Research & UK Key Advances
Series Organiser at St Bartholomew's Hospital, London*

UeL University Centre for
Public Health Policy &
Health Services Research

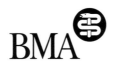

British Medical Association

British
Association of
Urological Surgeons

AESCULAPIUS MEDICAL PRESS
LONDON SAN FRANCISCO SYDNEY

Published by

Aesculapius Medical Press (London, San Francisco, Sydney)
Centre for Public Health Policy and Faculty of Science and Health
University of East London
33 Shore Road
London E9 7TA

First published 2000

British Library Cataloguing in Publication Data

A catalogue record for this book is available from the British Library

ISBN 1 903044 04 9

While the advice and information in this book are believed to be true and accurate at the
time of going to press, neither the authors nor the publishers nor the sponsoring institutions
can accept any legal responsibility or liability for any errors or omissions that may be made.
In particular (but without limiting the generality of the preceding disclaimer) every effort has
been made to check drug usages; however, it is possible that errors have been missed.
Furthermore, dosage schedules are constantly being revised and new side-effects recognised.
For these reasons, the reader is strongly urged to consult the drug companies' printed
instructions before administering any of the drugs recommended in this book.

Further copies of this volume are available from:

Claudio Melchiorri
Research Dissemination Fellow
Centre for Public Health Policy and Faculty of Science and Health
University of East London
33 Shore Road
London E9 7TA

Fax: 020 8525 8661

Typeset, printed and bound in Britain by
Peter Powell Origination & Print Limited

Contents

Contributors

Paul Abrams MD FRCS, Professor of Urology, Bristol Urological Institute, Southmead Hospital, Bristol

John Anderson ChM FRCS, Consultant Urological Surgeon, Royal Hallamshire Hospital, Sheffield

Richard Bell FRCS, Consultant Urological Surgeon, Northampton General Hospital, Northampton

Angela Billington RGN RM Dip HV, Specialist Nurse, North Herts Access Clinic, Baldock, Hertfordshire

Simon St Clair Carter MD FRCS, Consultant Urological Surgeon, Charing Cross Hospital, London

Michael Dineen FRCS, Consultant Urological Surgeon, Chelsea & Westminster Hospital, London

Mark Emberton MD FRCS (Urology), Senior Lecturer in Oncological Urology, Institute of Urology and Nephrology, University College, London, and Assistant Director, Clinical Effectiveness Unit, Royal College of Surgeons of England

Simon Fradd FRCS, Deputy Chairman, Joint General Practitioners Committee, The British Medical Association, London

Michael Kirby MB BS MRCP, General Practitioner, and Director of HertNet, The Hertfordshire Primary Care Research Network, University of Hertfordshire, Hatfield

David Kirk DM FRCS, Consultant Urologist, Gartnavel General Hospital, Glasgow, Scotland

Tom McNicholas MB BS FRCS FEBU, Consultant Urological Surgeon, Lister Hospital, Stevenage, Hertfordshire

Ronald A Miller MS FRCS, Consultant Director, Department of Minimally Invasive Surgery and Urology, Whittington Hospital, London

Richard J Simpson MB ChB DPM FRCPsych MRCGP, Forth Valley Primary Care Research Group, University of Stirling, Stirling, Scotland

Antony J Young FRCS, Research Fellow in Urology, University College, London and the Whittington Hospital, London

Preface

The progress in effective management of lower urinary tract symptoms (LUTS) related to benign prostatic disease (BPD) is one of the remarkable achievements of twentieth century medicine. Mortality from urinary outflow obstruction is now rare in the Western world and the morbidity of this group of conditions is now substantially reduced. However, while these are considerable achievements, there remain challenges, not least the choice of treatment for non-life threatening symptoms. When quality of life adjustments are the primary issue rather than mortality, then it is appropriate to review the standard surgical options and to explore the burgeoning alternatives, particularly the medical treatment options.

This volume explores current issues in the management of BPD/LUTS. A review of the epidemiology is fundamental to any reconsideration of the conditions and sets the scene for traditional hospital specialist-based management to be compared and contrasted to newer, community-based methods of assessment. Such methods may be suitable for most of the less severely obstructed or symptomatic men, but these new models of care still need critical analysis and probably adjustment in order to avoid deterioration in care for some men. Clearly, the current trend towards transfer of care (and presumably of funds) from secondary to primary care tends to encourage this process and the transfer needs to be guided by evidence.

Certain men will still need more formal and detailed 'specialist' assessment. This role is explored. Finally, in the process of diagnosis there remains the problem of excluding men with 'significant' prostate cancer, significant in the sense that the diagnosis might alter life expectancy or suggest different treatment options.

Having made an assessment, which treatment is to be offered? Patients, GPs (and specialists too) are surrounded by multiple options for both diagnosis and therapy. They can be forgiven for feeling uncertain as to the best option. Four chapters in this volume debate the evidence underpinning the competing claims for medical and surgical therapy for BPD/LUTS. As always, an update on the latest changes in the layout of the National Health Service in the UK is useful to alert us to the opportunities and threats that lie ahead.

In the current age, where doctors and health professionals are increasingly overwhelmed by clinical information, we have aimed to provide a fully current, fully referenced text which is as succinct as possible but as comprehensive as necessary. Consultants and training grades in urology and general practitioners will find it of particular use as part of continuing medical education and specialist training, and we advance it explicitly as an excellent tool for these purposes. We anticipate, however, that the book will prove of not inconsiderable use to other members of the primary health care team, hospital urology nurses and pharmacists as a reference text, and to commissioners of health services as the basis for discussion and negotiation of health contracts with their practising colleagues.

In conclusion, we thank Abbott Pharmaceuticals Ltd for the grant of educational sponsorship which helped organise a national symposium on BPD and LUTS at the British Medical Association, at which synopses of the constituent chapters of this book were presented.

Tom McNicholas MB BS FRCS FEBU
Michael Kirby MB BS MRCP
Andrew Miles MSc MPhil PhD

PART 1

Evidence and assessment

Epidemiological aspects of benign prostatic disease and lower urinary tract symptoms

Richard J Simpson

Introduction

The number of transurethral resections of the prostate (TURP) carried out in England rose from 10,000 in 1975 (National Hospital In Patient Enquiry (HIPE) data) to 37,000 in 1989–90 (National Hospital Episode (HES) data). This was probably due to decreasing mortality associated with TURP and demographic changes. But it is the renewed interest in benign prostatic hyperplasia (BPH) in the 1990s following the introduction of medical treatment that has led to the emergence in abundance of new epidemiological data. The first change was one in nomenclature from 'benign prostatic hypertrophy' to 'benign prostatic hyperplasia'.

Prevalence

Early population studies of BPH included those by Jensen *et al.* (1986) in Denmark and Wattanabe (1986) in Japan. These seemed to support anecdotal reports that BPH was a condition affecting older men, with about one in four men over 50 years being affected in some way.

Berry *et al.* (1984), reporting on a series of five necropsy studies, showed hyperplasia to exist almost exclusively in glands greater than 20 g and in men over 30 years of age. Necropsy studies do not necessarily reflect true community prevalence rates. However, in this case, further evidence from the Baltimore longitudinal study of ageing (Guess *et al.* 1990) showed a good level of agreement with autopsy prevalence rates.

This 'definition' of BPH as being glands over 20 g was employed in the first large community studies. In 1991 the Stirling BPH study group (Garraway *et al.* 1991) reported lower prevalence rates than the autopsy studies, but with rates of benign prostatic enlargement (BPE) in men increasing from 138 per 1,000 for those aged 40–49 to 430 for those aged 60–69. The widely quoted prevalence rate of one man in three over 50 years having BPH has largely stemmed from this study. However, these rates were derived only after selection of those men who, having been found to have either urinary flow rates of below 15 ml/sec or a level of lower urinary tract symptoms (LUTS) of more than 11 on the American Urological Association (AUA) scale or both, were referred for hospital-based transrectal ultrasound (TRUS). A parallel study, done in Omstead County, USA, by the Mayo Clinic (Chute *et al.* 1993), showed similar levels to the Scottish community study.

Only when an unselected community-based population was investigated by TRUS as a second phase of the study (Simpson *et al.* 1996) in Stirling, Scotland, were true rates of BPE determined. Much higher levels than previously were found, with the following distribution:

- age 40–49, 615 per thousand (95% CI 515–715)
- age 50–59, 776 per thousand (95% CI 688–865)
- age 60–69, 892 per thousand (95% CI 825–958)
- age 79–79, 889 per thousand (95% CI 744–1,000).

CI = Confidence Interval

BPE is now recognised to be so frequent as to be considered as much a normal part of ageing as grey hair or wrinkles (see Figure 1.1).

The problem surrounding agreement on a universal definition of BPH is only partially resolved and, without the clarity of a definition, the true prevalence rate in the community for the 'disease' of BPH remains uncertain.

In a seminal editorial in the *BMJ* Abrams (1994) proposed substitution of LUTS for 'prostatism'. LUTS could be combined with enlargement (BPE) and benign outlet obstruction (BOO) into what may become known as 'benign prostatic disease', represented by Hald's (1989) overlapping rings (see Figure 1.2).

Impact

An important element of this disease is its impact on the individual. Reporting on the impact on daily living activities in men aged 40–79, Garraway *et al.* (1993b) found that at least one out of the five following symptoms (nocturia twice or more, hesitancy, straining, intermittency and weak stream force) was reported as bothersome by twice as many men with BPH as those without – the largest differences being for urgency and intermittency. Forty-seven per cent of men with BPH reporting four or more symptoms also found them bothersome compared with 16 per cent of men without BPH. Garraway *et al.* went on to extrapolate the data to suggest that no fewer than half a million men in the UK of working age were affected in at least one activity of daily living most or all of the time, demonstrating a substantial unmet need.

Men adapt their lives to accommodate urinary symptoms: one in three men curtail their fluid intake before bed or before travelling.

Consultation patterns and attitudes

The Stirling study also found that, after controlling for age, men with moderate symptoms were six times more likely to consult their general practitioner than men with mild symptoms (odds ratio 6.1, 95% CI 3.9–9.4) (Simpson *et al.* 1994). But overall men who were experiencing symptoms and indeed bothersomeness did not consult to any great extent.

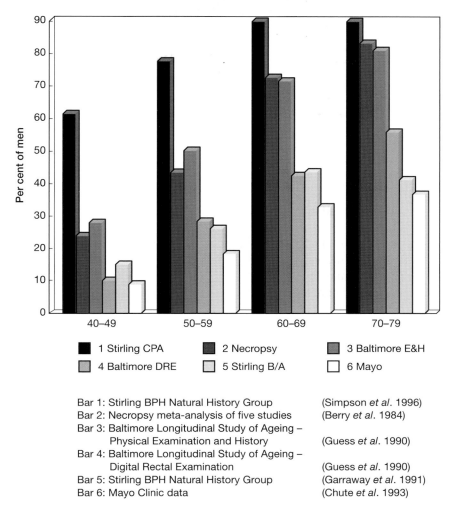

Bar 1: Stirling BPH Natural History Group (Simpson *et al*. 1996)
Bar 2: Necropsy meta-analysis of five studies (Berry *et al*. 1984)
Bar 3: Baltimore Longitudinal Study of Ageing –
        Physical Examination and History (Guess *et al*. 1990)
Bar 4: Baltimore Longitudinal Study of Ageing –
        Digital Rectal Examination (Guess *et al*. 1990)
Bar 5: Stirling BPH Natural History Group (Garraway *et al*. 1991)
Bar 6: Mayo Clinic data (Chute *et al*. 1993)

Source: (Adapted with permission of H Guess)

Figure 1.1. Age-specific prevalence of benign prostatic hyperplasia

Two studies have indicated possible reasons for this failure to consult. The first by Boyle (1994), a European study on attitudes, suggested that the main fear men had in relation to prostate disease was about cancer. Cunningham-Burley *et al*. (1996) in a qualitative study found that the insidious development of symptoms led to their acceptance as part of the normal ageing process. Men's perceptions were that a prostatic 'illness' would cause pain or haematuria or acute retention. Indeed, 75 per cent of the men in this study who had undergone prostatectomy had presented with

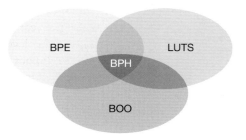

BPH: Benign Prostatic Hyperplasia
BPE: Benign Prostatic Enlargement
BOO: Bladder Outflow Obstruction
LUTS: Lower Urinary Tract Symptoms

Source: Hald (1989)

Figure 1.2 Benign prostatic hyperplasia – a definition

one or more of these symptoms. A finding of some importance to clinicians was that bothersomeness was not synonymous with worry or problem. The interference with daily living activities may 'bother' but is not perceived as significant or alarming enough to consult a doctor.

The MORI poll in 1993 (Brocklehurst 1993) suggested that in cases of urinary incontinence from any cause, 52 per cent of men consulted a doctor and were not embarrassed to consult. In a more recent poll (Men's Health Matters/Gallup survey 1997) many more men seemed to be aware of the prostate and problems associated with it. The findings indicate a shift in attitudes, with 91 per cent of men reporting they were not embarrassed about consulting a doctor and 40 per cent of older men with problems claiming to have actually consulted a doctor in the previous year.

The Stirling follow-up study confirmed baseline findings and the findings of the Omstead County cohort. Men were more likely to consult the worse their symptom score.

Progression

The symptoms which patients experience are thought not to progress over time in many instances. Follow-up studies by Birkhoff *et al.* (1976) showed half the patients unchanged or improved over a two-year period (n=26). Ball *et al.* (1981) followed up 127 men with prostatism, for five years, of whom 97 remained untreated. There was an assumption, not dispelled by these earlier studies, that men with problems would deteriorate at least at a faster rate than those who had no problems. The Stirling BPH Natural History Group found in the much larger sample, followed over one year (Garraway *et al.* 1993a), three years (Lee *et al.* 1996) and five years (Lee *et al.* 1998b), that the overall prevalence of urinary symptoms increased in all three follow-up periods for the group as a whole. Of those men found to have urgency and dribbling at the outset of the study, up to a quarter improved at the one-year review, while only one third reported urinary symptoms to have deteriorated. The levels of bothersomeness to these men, caused by their urinary symptoms, also did not show much change in the first year. There was an overall increase of 19 per cent in urinary peak flow in the first year. Such increases may be due to familiarisation (Posnanski & Posnanski 1969), though this is mainly demonstrated in younger men (Dutarte & Susset 1974). There is a general decline in uroflow with ageing (Jensen *et al.* 1987) shown in normative age-related data sets (Haylen *et al.* 1989).

At three-year follow-up (Lee *et al.* 1996) of the Stirling cohort, 224 (95 per cent) out of 256 men aged 40–79 with BPE reported an increase in the overall level of interference with selected daily living activities. Compared with base levels, men in the cohort as a whole who reported interference with at least one activity of daily living increased from 49 to 63 per cent, and those with three activities affected increased from 21 to 28 per cent. However, the pattern of change showed considerable within-subject variation, with almost as many men improving as deteriorating.

At five years, with 71 per cent (n=1,177/1,994 now aged 45–84 years) of the original Stirling cohort respondents still participating in the study, a review was again undertaken of the symptoms and bothersomeness and interference with activities of daily living (Lee *et al.* 1998b). This showed a continuing deterioration in LUTS and bothersomeness for the group as a whole from baseline to five years. The largest increases were in straining, hesitancy, incomplete emptying, weak stream and nocturia. This was at some variance from the Omstead County 42-month follow-up (Jacobsen *et al.* 1996), which had found that weak stream, nocturia, dribbling and wet clothes showed the largest annual change.

The increase in bothersomeness of dribbling, incomplete emptying, weak stream, frequency, nocturia and intermittency was more pronounced than the increase in the prevalence or mean for all symptoms. On the other hand, the increase in interference in levels of selected activities of daily living arising from LUTS was less marked.

The progression of LUTS over time in individual men was very variable, a finding mirroring that of a four-year follow-up in the USA (Barry *et al.* 1997). Of 500 candidates for TURP presenting to US urological practices, who were treated non-operatively, there were 371 survivors with complete data at four years. Of 60 men with mild, 245 with moderate and 66 with severe symptoms, 10, 24 and 39 per cent respectively had undergone TURP; 27, 31 and 27 per cent respectively were on pharmacological treatment; and 63, 45 and 33 per cent respectively were not on active treatment.

Although the gradual deterioration of the Stirling group as a whole from the initial baseline findings at one-year, three-year and five-year reviews was predictable, the continued and sustained improvement in a minority of men at five years was unexpected. The findings of all three cohort studies lend substantial support to the likely long-term benefit of both 'watchful waiting' and medical treatment modalities.

The studies in Stirling, Scotland and Ohmstead County, USA, are likely to be the last community cohort studies undertaken and their continuation is of considerable importance to our knowledge of BPH.

Uroflow

Normative data combining ageing, voided volume and uroflow have been attempted (Drach *et al.* 1979; Haylen *et al.* 1989; Jacobsen *et al.* 1996; Barry *et al.* 1997) but their value is questionable (Jorgensen *et al.* 1986). Although Qmax is generally accepted as the key indicator (Jensen 1989), it is not, of itself, sufficient to diagnose BOO. Uroflow is the product of bladder contractions and urethral capacity. It can be affected by stricture and by abdominal straining as well as psychological stress (Jensen 1995). Variations within individuals of 4.1 ml/sec or more have been observed and, for this reason, paired readings may be valuable (Barry *et al.* 1995c). Regression to the mean, found in repeated measures in a cohort selected originally for low Qmax, emphasises the dangers of isolated uroflow readings in diagnosing BPH (Prescott & Garraway 1995). Despite these caveats it would appear that Qmax readings of >20 ml/sec are unlikely to be associated with BPE of >40 g and Qmax can therefore be used as an indication of prostate size (Simpson *et al.* 1996). A prostate-specific antigen (PSA) of less than 2 ng/ml is another alternative marker for smaller prostates.

Symptom scores

Barry *et al.* (1995b) underlined the benefits of using validated instruments such as the AUA Symptom Index (Barry *et al.* 1992) and the IPSS Symptom Index, which have an additional specific 'quality of life' question. The IPSS is widely used in Europe, though there are some doubts about its validity in all languages. The earlier Boyarsky Index (Boyarsky *et al.* 1977) was developed for evaluative rather than predictive purposes, whereas the Madsen-Iversen Index (Madsen-Iversen 1983) was designed to aid selection of patients for surgical intervention. While symptom score can help to underpin the clinical evaluation, it is important to recognise at the outset that higher scores on many of these symptom indices do not diagnose BPH, nor even distinguish adequately between BOO, bladder neck or urethral stricture (Chancellor *et al.* 1994). Indeed such scores may be achieved by women (Lepor & Machi 1993)! The increasing importance of the impact of LUTS upon a patient's quality of life has been recognised by the introduction in the USA of a questionnaire on 'troublesomeness' (Barry *et al.* 1995a), which will need further evaluation in the UK. This Symptom Problem Index includes the following four questions:

- How much physical discomfort did the urinary problems cause?
- How much worry did the patient have because of urinary problems?
- How bothersome was the urination over the past month?
- How much time had the problems kept the patient from doing the kind of things he would usually do?

However, in the first published community application of the impact scale in the UK (Lee *et al.* 1998b) it has not proved as robust as was expected.

Correlation of LUTS, prostate size and uroflow

Two community-based studies reported by Girman *et al.* (1995) from the Omstead County cohort in the USA, and Bosch *et al.* (1995) in a Dutch study showed a number of weak correlations. These were between IPSS scores and prostate volume (0.185 and 0.19 p<0.001); between prostate volume and peak urinary flow rate (-0.214 and 0.18 p<0.001); and between IPSS scores and peak urinary flow (-0.35 and -0.18 p<0.001). Most recently, Lee *et al.* (1998a) reporting on the Stirling cohort at baseline and at three-year follow-up failed to demonstrate any relationship other than between prostate volume and nocturia (n=193, r=0.202, p=0.0057). Furthermore, the weak correlations which were demonstrated accounted for only 9 per cent of the total variation of prostate or adenoma volume or their dimensions. In reviewing the evidence available up to the fourth International Consultation on BPH in Paris in July 1997, the committee on epidemiology, under the chairmanship of Oishi, suggested that although only weak correlations were to be found, they may be as clinically significant as the relationship between cholesterol and coronary artery occlusion (r=0.15) (Oishi 1997).

Risk factors

Biochemical

Dihydrotestosterone plays a central role in the development of the prostate (Imperato-McGinley 1974), but the biochemical factors underlying enlargement associated with increasing age are unclear. Current thinking (Colombel *et al.* 1998) suggests that BPE may be due to an increasing imbalance between factors associated with cell growth or proliferation and those associated with cell death (apoptosis). Clearly, understanding of the interplay between the various growth factors may lead to the development of newer and better medical treatments (Habib 1995).

Racial, social and demographic factors

Guess (1992) summarised the published evidence with respect to racial, social and geographical variation in BPH as 'fragmentary, partly based on anecdotal reports and limited by a lack of structural diagnostic criteria and modes of case ascertainment'. The problem with many of the studies to date is that they employ TURP as a marker for BPH and we know that the decision to undergo operation especially in the USA is a matter of patient choice (since most operations are for symptoms rather than absolute indications).

Smoking

Moderate smoking may be associated with lower rates of prostatectomy (Morrison 1978; Roberts *et al.* 1994). This may be as much due to early death or unfitness for elective surgery in older male smokers as to any possible causal relationship with BPH (Glynn *et al.* 1985). Roberts *et al.* (1994) in analysing data from the Mayo cohort study of 2,115 men showed a biphasic response to smoking, with light smokers having a decreased risk of LUTS and heavy smokers an increased risk. An elegant hypothesis for these findings was that lower levels of smoking improved bladder function, hence the decreased risk. However, the study was flawed due to the cross-sectional nature of the design and the comparatively low level of smokers (16 per cent) in the sample. Roberts himself went on to conduct a similar study in 286 Japanese men (Roberts *et al.* 1997) which showed similar overall results. Smokers are less likely to have flow rates of <15 ml/sec and prostate volumes of >40 ml. But the Japanese men who were light smokers showed an increase and not a decrease in LUTS. Kupeli (1997) found a larger mean prostate volume in non-smokers but found no enzymatic mechanisms to account for the apparent effect of smoking. The conclusion at present must be that there is no clear relationship and no tenable hypothesis for any such relationship.

Alcohol/cirrhosis

Evidence for a relationship between BPH and cirrhosis (Stumph & Willen 1953) is also equivocal. However, there may be an inverse association between alcohol consumption and eventual prostatectomy (Chyou *et al.* 1993), but as with smoking, this may be due to earlier death of high alcohol consumption patients (Araki *et al.* 1983). More direct evidence comes from studies such as the Kyoto study reported by Nukui (1997) where a negative risk of BPH was found to be related to alcohol consumption.

Dietary factors

A study reviewing BPH in rural, as opposed to urban, China (Gu 1997) has suggested that increasing prevalence could be attributed to increases in daily intake of total calories, fat and animal protein and decreased daily intake of vegetables and whole grain. Nukui (1997), on the other hand, concluded that increased ingestion of betacarotene was associated with increased risks of BPH. Until there are clearer causal relationships, the role of diet will also be debatable.

Social class

Early reports (Richardson 1964; Araki *et al.* 1983) that BPH was more prevalent in those with higher educational backgrounds or social class were found, but in studies flawed by highly selected populations. The Stirling community study (Simpson *et al.* 1994) found no social class variation. Evidence from Emberton *et al.* (1995) of higher rates of TURP, in patients with moderate symptoms, in the private sector, confirms the probable bias of the earlier studies.

Family history/genetic factors

Genetic factors appear to play some part, as shown both in twin studies (Partin *et al.* 1994) and in case control studies (Sanda *et al.* 1994). However, the association of BPH with a reported family history of BPH is unclear. Roberts *et al.* (1995) reported on 440 out of 2,119 men indicating a family history of enlarged prostate in a community study. After correction both for age and for degree of urological worry, the findings were significant (odds ratio 1.3, 95 per cent CI 1.0–1.6). This study also found that the risks were greater for those men whose relatives had been diagnosed at a younger age (odds ratio 2.5, 95 per cent CI 1.5–4.3).

Examining the extensive database created from the Merck phase III finasteride clinical trial, Sanda *et al.* (1997) reviewed 69 men who had familial BPH (three or more members in a family with BPH). The mean prostate size of this subgroup was 82.7 ml compared to 55.5 ml of the control group of 345 men with no family history (p<0.001). Men with this level of family clustering have a frequency of 46 per cent in the largest decile of prostate size and only 13 per cent in the smallest decile. The conclusion was that a genetic factor responsible for familial growth might exert its influence through androgen-independent control of prostatic growth. There would appear to be further scope for research in this area.

Sexual function

Neither the Stirling study nor the Omstead County study quoted above resulted in adequate data on sexual functioning. However, Frankel *et al.* (1998) reviewed both community attendees (n=423) in the UK and urologic clinic attendees (n=1,271) aged 45 years and over in 12 countries. LUTS were found to be strongly associated with sexual dysfunction independent of ageing. Moreover many older men remained markedly concerned about this dysfunction. This study confirmed an earlier report on French men aged over 50 years (MacFarlane *et al.* 1996).

Although in 'best practice' men's sexual function is reviewed as part of pre-operative assessment, this is neither universal nor even common in assessing quality of life issues before assigning patients to watchful waiting or medical treatment.

Male pattern baldness

Anecdotal evidence of an association between male pattern baldness and BPH was given credence in 1998 by a case control study from South Korea by Oh *et al.* (1998) in which men over 60 years with BPH had a greater proportion, with a higher grade of androgenic alopecia (54 versus 37 per cent p<0.01) and greater frequency of inherited baldness (32 versus 13 per cent p<0.001).

Physical activity

In the continuing search for associations with lifestyle factors that may lessen the impact of natural BPE, diet has already been mentioned. Comparison was made between men who had a TURP (n=1,890) or developed LUTS (n=1,853) scoring more than 15 and men who scored less than 7 on the AUA symptom score (n=21,745). These men were followed up over 8 years (1986–94). This study (Platz et al. 1998) showed evidence of an inverse relationship between physical activity and both BPH (odds ratio 0.75, 95 per cent CI 0.67–0.85) and TURP (odds ratio 0.76, 95 per cent CI 0.64–0.90). It is not yet clear how these new data fit with previous contradictory studies of obesity (Glynn et al. 1985; Daniell 1993).

Complications

Urinary retention

Almost 30 per cent of men who go on to have prostatectomy present with acute urinary retention (US Department of Health & Human Sciences 1994; Emberton et al. 1995). Birkhoff et al. (1976) felt this presentation to be independent of the degree of prostatism (n=26). In an East Anglian practice, Craigen et al. (1969) found a mean reported symptom duration of less than three months in acute retention (n=89) and following up those (n=129) who had not presented in this way, found less than 10 per cent developing acute retention over the next seven years. Powell et al. (1980), who found little evidence of symptoms warning of retention, replicated these findings. In the Omstead County cohort study in a follow-up of 8,344 person-years Jacobsen et al. (1997a) reported on the occurrence of urinary retention. A rate of 6.8/1,000 person-years was found (95 per cent CI 5.2–8.9).

Boyle (1998) reviewed our current knowledge of the epidemiology of urinary retention in 1998. It is now clear that this unpleasant experience often leading to admission is common. The risks would appear to have a probability of about 23 per cent over the next 20 years in men aged 60 if they survive. The risk of this event rises with age and will occur more frequently in men with moderate or severe LUTS and in men with low flow rates (<12 ml/sec) and larger prostates. Kurita et al. (1998) has suggested the transitional zone (TZ) index (TZ volume/total prostate volume) as a refinement to simple prostate volume as a risk indicator. Although this requires further work, it is an interesting concept.

Renal

BOO can lead to recurrent urinary tract infection and pyelonephritis or chronic urinary retention, dilatation and hydronephrosis. Acute renal failure reported by Feest et al. (1993) as having an incidence of 172 per million adults yearly, noted that in 25 per cent (31/125) of the patients this was due to prostatic disease. This prostate group had a survival rate, which was not age-related, of 84 per cent at three months. Chronic renal failure, where prostatic causation accounts for a lesser proportion, perhaps 12 per cent (Kaufman et al. 1991), may be entirely preventable (Sack et al. 1989) and should be detected by general practitioners (Cairns & Woolfson 1994).

Elevated urea/creatinine is associated with precipitant admission (Emberton *et al.* 1995) with the patient more likely in the UK to be operated on by trainees. Such elevations are associated with more post-operative complications and mortality (Holtgrewe & Walk 1962; Melchior *et al.* 1974; Mebust *et al.* 1989).

Bladder stones

Bladder stones were reported as a reason for prostatectomy in 1–2 per cent of cases (Doll *et al.* 1992; Thorpe *et al.* 1994; US Department of Health & Human Sciences 1994; Emberton *et al.* 1995). Grosse (1980) in a large necropsy study (n=19,863) found the prevalence of stones in men over the age of 60 at a rate eight times higher in those with BPE (3.4 per cent) than in either non-BPE men (0.4 per cent) or women (0.3 per cent). The Omstead County cohort study in their 8,344 person-years follow-up found a rate of kidney stones of 6.0/1,000 person-years, 50 men in all.

Conclusions

The past decade has seen an explosion of epidemiological information on BPH. The main conclusions that can be drawn from all this new evidence are that BPE is almost universal in older men. It is also clear that the impact on the quality of men's lives was previously largely unrecognised. The condition is now better understood both in terms of its symptomatology and its progression. The rates of complications are now being enumerated and some of the risk factors are becoming defined. However, the 14 recommendations for epidemiological research which emerged from the 1997 WHO-sponsored consultaton on BPH (Jacobsen *et al.* 1997b) remain largely valid. In particular, there is still a need for a working epidemiological definition of BPH and LUTS.

References

Abrams P (1994). New words for old, lower urinary tract symptoms for 'prostatism' [editorial]. *BMJ* **308**, 929–30.

Araki H, Wattanabe H, Mishina T & Nakao M (1983). High risk group for BPH. *The Prostate* **4**, 253–64.

Ball AJ, Fenelly RCL & Abrams PH (1981). The natural history of untreated prostatism. *Br J Urol* **53**, 613–16.

Barry MJ, Fowler FJ, O'Leary MP *et al.* (1992). The American Urological Association Symptom Index for benign prostatic hyperplasia. *J Urol* **148**, 1549–57.

Barry MJ, Floyd FJ, O'Leary MP, Bruskewitz RC, Holtgrewe HL, Mebust WK & the Measurement Committee of the American Urological Association (1995a). Measuring disease-specific health status in men with BPH. *APHA Medical Care* section Suppl. **4/33**(4), 144–55.

Barry MJ, Fowler FJ, O'Leary MP, Bruskewitz RC, Holtgrew HL, Meburst WK & the Measurement Committee of the American Urological Association (1995b). Measuring disease-specific health status in men with BPH. *Med Care* **33**(4)(Suppl.), 145–55.

Barry MJ, Girman CJ, O'Leary M *et al.* (1995c). Using repeated measures of symptom score, uroflow and PSA in the clinical management of prostate disease. *J Urol* **153**, 99–103.

Barry MJ, Fowler FJ Jr, Bin L, Pitts JC III, Harris CJ & Mulley AG Jr (1997). The natural history of patients with BPH as diagnosed by North American urologists. *J Urol* **157**, 10–15.

Berry SJ, Coffey DS, Walsh PC & Ewing LL (1984). The development of human benign prostatic hyperplasia with age. *J Urol* **132**, 474–9.

Birkhoff JD, Weiderhorn AR, Hamilton ML & Zinsser HH (1976). Natural history of BPH (hypertrophy) and acute urinary retention. *J Urol* **7**, 48–52.

Bosch JLHR, Hop WCJ, Kirkels WJ & Schroeder FH (1995). The IPSS in a community-based sample of men between 55–74 years of age, prevalence and correlation of symptoms with age prostate volume, flow rate and residual urine. *Br J Urol* **75**, 622–30.

Boyarsky S, Jones G, Paulson DF & Prou GR Jr (1977). New look at bladder neck obstruction by food and drug administration regulators; guidelines for investigations of BPH. *Transactions of AMA of GU Surgeons* **68**, 29–32.

Boyle P (1994). New insights into the epidemiology and natural history of BPH. *Prog Clin Biol Res* **386**, 3–18.

Boyle P (1998). Some remarks on the epidemiology of acute urinary retention. *Arch Ital Androl* **70**(2), 77–82.

Brocklehurst JC, on behalf of the British Association for Continence Care (1993). Urinary incontinence in the community – analysis of a MORI poll. *BMJ* **306**, 832–4.

Cairns HS & Woolfson RG (1994). Prevention of end stage renal failure, an achievable goal [editorial]. *Br J Gen Pract* Nov, 486.

Chancellor MB, Rivas DA, Keeley FX, Lofti MA & Gomella LG (1994). Similarity of AUA Symptom Index among men with BPH and detrusor hyperreflexia without BOO. *Br J Urol* **74**, 200–3.

Chute CG, Panser LA, Johnson CL *et al.* (1993). The prevalence of prostatism, a population based survey of urinary symptoms. *J Urol* **150**, 85–9.

Chyou PH, Nomura AMY, Stemmerman GN & Hankin JH (1993). A prospective study of alcohol, diet, and other lifestyle factors in relation to obstructive uropathy. *Prostate* **22**, 253–64.

Colombel M, Vacherot F, Diez SG, Fontaine E, Buttyan R & Chopin D (1998). Zonal variation of apoptosis and proliferation in the normal prostate and in BPH. *B J Urol* **82**, 380–5.

Craigen AA, Hickling JB, Saunders CRG & Carpenter RG (1969). *J R Coll Gen Practit* **18**, 226–32.

Cunningham-Burley S, Allbutt H, Garraway WM, Lee AJ & Russell BAW (1996). Perceptions of urinary symptoms and health care seeking behaviour amongst men aged 40–79. *B J Gen Pract* **46**, 349–52.

Daniell HW (1993). More stage A prostatic cancers, less surgery for BPH in smokers. *J Urol* **149**, 68–72.

Doll HA, Black NA, McPherson MC, Flood AB, Williams GB & Smith JC (1992). Mortality, morbidity and complications following TURP for BPH (hypertrophy). *J Urol* **147**, 1566–73.

Drach GW, Layton TN & Binard WJ (1979). Male peak urinary flow rate, relationship to voided volume and age. *J Urol* **122**, 210–14.

Dutarte D & Susset JG (1974). Reproducibilite des courbes de debitmetrie urinaire. *J Urol Nephrol (Paris)* **80**, 484–94.

Emberton M, Neal DE, Black N, Harrison M, Fordham M, McBrian MP, Williams RE, McPherson K & Devlin HB (1995). The national prostatectomy audit, the clinical management of patients during hospital admission. *Br J Urol* **75**, 301–16.

Feest TG, Round A & Hamad S (1993). Incidence of severe renal failure in adults, results of a community based study. *BMJ* **306**, 481–3.

Frankel SJ, Donovan JL, Peters TI, Dabhoiwala NF, Osawa D & Lin AT (1998). Sexual dysfunction in men with LUTS. *J Clin Epidemiol* **51**(8), 677–85.

Garraway WM, Collins GW & Lee RJ (1991). High prevalence of benign prostatic hypertrophy in the community. *Lancet* **338**, 469–71.

Garraway WM, Armstrong C, Auld S, King D & Simpson RJ (1993a). Follow-up of a cohort of men with untreated BPH. *Eur Urol* **24**, 313–18.

Garraway WM, Russell EBAW, Lee RJ, Collins GN, Mckelvie GB, Hehir M, Rogers ACN & Simpson RJ (1993b). Impact of previously unrecognised BPH on the daily activities of middle aged and elderly men. *B J Gen Prac* **43**, 318–21.

Girman CJ, Jacobsen SJ, Guess HA, Oesterling JE, Chute CG, Panser LA & Lieber MM (1995). Natural history of prostatism. Relationship among symptoms, prostate size and peak urinary flow rate. *J Urol* **153**, 1510–15.

Glynn RJ, Campion EW, Bouchard GR *et al.* (1985). The development of BPH amongst volunteers in the normative ageing study. *Am J Epid* **121**, 78–90.

Grosse H (1980). Frequency, localisation and associated disorders in urinary calculi. *Z Urol Nephrol* **83**, 469–74.

Gu F (1997). Changes in the prevalence of BPH in China. *Chin Med (Engl)* **110**(3), 163–6.

Guess HA (1992). *BPH antecedents and natural history; epidemiological review.* Vol. 14. John Hopkins University School of Hygiene and Public Health.

Guess HA, Arrighi HM, Metter EJ *et al.* (1990). Cumulative prevalence of prostatism matches the autopsy prevalence of BPH. *Prostate* **17**, 241–6.

Habib FK (1995). Hormonal influences on the prostate gland. In *Epidemiology of prostate disease* (ed. WM Garraway), Chapter 2. Springer Verlag, New York.

Hald T (1989). Urodynamics in BPH, a survey. *Prostate* Suppl. **2**, 69–77

Haylen BT, Ashby D, Sutherst JR, Frazer MI & West CR (1989). Maximum and average urine flow rates in normal male and female populations – the Liverpool nomograms. *Br J Urol* **64**, 30–8.

Holtgrewe HL & Walk WL. Factors influencing the mortality and morbidity of TURP: a study of 2,015 cases. *J Urol* **112**, 634–42.

Imperato-McGinley J, Guerrero L, Gautier T *et al.* (1974). Steroid 5-alpha-reductase deficiency in man, an inherited form of male pseudohermaphroditism. *Science* **186**, 1213–15.

Jacobsen SJ, Girman CJ, Guess HA, Rhodes T, Oesterling JE & Lieber MM (1996). Natural history of prostatism. Longitudinal changes in voiding symptoms in community dwelling men. *J Urol* **155**, 595–600.

Jacobsen SJ, Jacobsen DJ, Girman CJ, Roberts RO, Rhodes T, Guess HA & Leiber MM (1997a). Natural history of prostatism, risk factors for urinary retention. *J Urol* **158**, 481–7.

Jacobsen SJ, Jacobsen DJ, Girman CJ, Roberts RO, Rhodes T, Guess HA & Leiber MM (1997b). Natural history of prostatism, urologic complications in community dwelling men. *JGIM* **12** (Suppl. 1), 53.

Jensen KM-E (1989). Clinical evaluaton of routine urodynamic investigations in prostatism. *Neurology and Urodynamics* **8**, 545–78.

Jensen KM-E (1995). Uroflowmetry in epidemiological studies of prostate disease, some critical considerations. In *Epidemiology of prostate disease* (ed. WM Garraway), pp.42–51. Springer Verlag, New York.

Jensen KM-E, Jorgensen JB, Morgansen P *et al.* (1986). Some clinical aspects of uroflowmetry in elderly males – a population study. *Scand J Urol Nephrol* **20**, 93–7.

Jensen KM-E, Jorgensen JB & Mogensen P (1987). Relationship between urinary flow curve patterns and symptomatology in elderly males. *Scand J Urol Nephrol* Suppl. **104**, 69–71.

Jorgensen JB, Jensen KM-E, Bille Brahe NE & Mogensen P (1986). Uroflowmetry in asymptomatic elderly males. *Br J Urol* **58**, 390–5.

Kaufman J, Dhakal M, Patel B *et al.* (1991). Community acquired acute renal failure. *Am J Kidney Dis* **17**, 191–8.

Kupeli B, Soygur T, Aydos K, Ozdiler E & Kupeli S (1997). The role of cigarette smoking in BPE. *Br J Urol* **80**(2), 201–4.

Kurita Y, Masuda H, Terada H, Suzuki K & Fujita K (1998). Transition zone index as a risk factor for acute urinary retention. *Urol* **51**(4), 595–600.

Lee AJ, Russell EBAW, Garraway WM & Prescott RJ (1996). Three-year follow up of a community based cohort of men with untreated BPH. *Eur Urol* **30**, 11–17.

Lee AJ, Garraway WM & Simpson RJ (1998a). Pathophysiological relationships between LUTS and the prostate do not strengthen over time. *Prostate* **37**, 5–9.

Lee AJ, Garraway WM, Simpson RJ, Fisher W & King D (1998b). The natural history of untreated LUTS in middle-aged and elderly men over a period of five years. *Eur Urol* **34**(4), 325–32.

Lepor H & Machi G (1993). Comparison of AUA symptom index in unselected males and females between 55 and 79 years of age. *Urol* **42**, 36–40.

Macfarlane G, Segnier PP, Botto H, Teillac P, Richard F & Boyle P (1996). *Relationship between LUTS and sexual life of French men over 50 years.* Abstracts AUA Congress, p. 233.

Madsen-Iversen P (1983). A point system for selecting operative candidates. In *Benign prostatic hypertrophy* (ed. S Boyarski & F Hinman), p.3. Springer Verlag, New York.

Mebust WK, Holtgrewe HL, Cockett ATK, Peters PC & writing committee (1989). TURP, immediate and post-operative complications. A cooperative study of 13 participating institutions evaluating 3,885 patients. *J Urol* **141**, 243–7.

Melchior J, Walk WL, Foret JD *et al.* (1974). Transurethral prostatectomy, computerised analysis of 2,223 consecutive cases. *Br J Urol* **112**, 634–42.

Men's Health Matters/Gallup survey (1997). A report.

Morrison AS (1978). Prostatic hypertrophy in Greater Boston. *J Chron Dis* **31**, 357–62.

National Hospital Episode (HES) data, 1989–1990.

National Hospital In Patient Enquiry (HIPE) data, 1975–1985.

Nukui M (1997). Epidemiological study on diet, smoking and alcohol drinking in the relationship to prostatic weight. *Nippon Hinyokika Gakkai Zasshi* **88**(11), 950–6.

Oh BR, Kim SJ, Moon JD, Kim HN, Kwon DD, Won YH, Ryu SB & Park YI (1998). Association of BPH with male pattern baldness. *Urol* **51**(5), 744–8.

Oishi K (1997). Epidemiology and natural history of BPH. In *Proceedings of the 4th International Consultation on BPH* (ed. L Denis, K Griffiths, S Khoury *et al.*), p.34. Health Publications Ltd.

Partin AW, Page WF, Lee BR, Sanda MG, Miller RN & Walsh PC (1994). Concordance rates for BPH among twins suggest hereditary influence. *Urology* **44**(5), 646–50.

Platz EA, Kawachi I, Rimm EB, Colditz GA, Stampfer MJ, Willett WC & Giovannucci E (1998). Physical activity and BPH. *Arch Intern Med* **158**(21), 2349–56.

Posnanski E & Posnanski AK (1969). Psychogenic influences on voiding – observations from voiding cystourethrography. *Psychosomatics* **10**, 339–42.

Powell PH, Smith PJ & Fenely RC (1980). The identification of patients at risk from acute retention. *Br J Urol* **52**, 520–2.

Prescott RJ & Garraway WM (1995). Regression to the mean occurs in measuring peak urinary flow. *Br J Urol* **76**, 611–13.

Richardson IM (1964). Prostatic hyperplasia and social class. *Br J Prev Soc Med* **18**, 157–62.

Roberts RO, Jacobsen SJ, Rhodes T, Guess HA, Girman CJ, Panser LA, Chute CG, Oesterling JE & Lieber MM (1994). Cigarette smoking and prostatism, a biphasic relation? *J Urol* **43**, 797–801.

Roberts RO, Rhodes T, Panser LA, Girman CJ, Chute CG, Guess HA, Oesterling JE, Lieber MM & Jacobsen SJ (1995). Association between family history of BPH and urinary symptoms, results of a population-based study. *Am J Epidemiol* **142**, 965–73.

Roberts RO, Tsukamoto T & Kumamoto Y (1997). Association between cigarette smoking and prostatism in a Japanese community. *Prostate* **30**, 154–9.

Sack SH, Aparicio SAJR, Bevin A *et al.* (1989). Late renal failure due to prostatic outflow obstruction, a preventable disease. *BMJ* **298**, 156–9.

Sanda MG, Beaty TH, Stutzman RE, Childs B & Walsh PC (1994). Genetic susceptibility of BPH. *J Urol* **152**, 115–19.

Sanda MG, Doerhing CB, Binkowitz B, Beaty TH, Partin AW, Hale E, Stoner E & Walsh (1997). Primary care. Clinical and biological characteristics of familial BPH. *J Urol* **157**(3), 876–9.

Simpson RJ (1997). BPH (review). *B J Gen Pract* **47**, 111–18.

Simpson RJ, Lee RJ, Garraway WM, King D & McIntosh I (1994). Consultation patterns in a community survey of men with BPH. *B J Gen Pract* **44**, 499–502.

Simpson RJ, Fisher, Lee AJ, Garraway M & Russell B (1996). Benign prostatic hyperplasia in an unselected, community based population. *B J Urol* **77**, 186–91.

Stumph HH & Willens SL (1953). Inhibitory effects of portal cirrhosis of the liver on prostatic enlargement. *Arch Int Med* **91**, 304–9.

Thorpe AC, Cleary R, Coles J, Vernon S, Reynolds J & Neal DE (1994). Deaths and complications following prostatectomy in 1400 men in the Northern Regional Prostate Audit Group. *Br J Urol* **74**, 559–65.

US Department of Health & Human Sciences (1994). *BPH, diagnosis and treatment. Clinical practice guidelines*. AHCPR Pub. No. 94–0582, Feb.

Wattanabe H (1986). A natural history of benign prostatic hypertrophy. *Ultrasound Med Biol* **12**, 567–71.

Chapter 2

Investigation and assessment: traditional versus innovative models of care

Michael Dineen, Tom McNicholas, Michael Kirby and Angela Billington

The treatment of BPH: an historical perspective

Herophilus (c.300 BC), the founder of the great medical school at Alexandria, is credited with first using the word 'prostate'. Little other reference is found to the gland until the mid-sixteenth century when Niccoló Masso (1536) of Padua mentions it again. Leonardo Da Vinci (1452–1519) in his drawings of the male urogenital tract completely ignores the prostate. Ambrose Pare in 1564 described the symptom complex, now recognised as that secondary to bladder outflow obstruction due to benign prostatic hyperplasia; he, however, attributed the outflow obstruction to carnosities of the bladder neck compounded by the weak expulsive efforts of the elderly. Jean Riolan (1577–1657) first suggested that the enlarged prostate may be the cause of symptoms. In 1788, John Hunter described prostatic enlargement and the deleterious effects this may have on the bladder and the upper tracts (Shelly 1969).

Catheterisation was for many centuries the only treatment for lower urinary tract symptoms (LUTS) and indeed metal catheters were found in the ashes of Vesuvius. The lack of medical interest until relatively recently is probably related to short life expectancy, with few men reaching an age where they were likely to be troubled by urinary symptoms. Pare is considered the father of transurethral surgery as he developed a device used to blindly ensnare prostatic tissue with a wire and shave it off. He believed that resulting haemorrage was beneficial to the patient as it relieved the congestion and allowed excess humours to escape. Seventeenth-century surgeons were experienced lithotomists frequently removing bladder stones, which were presumably due to a combination of diet and bladder outflow obstruction. Little progress was made until the development of prostatectomy approximately 100 years ago, although Philip Syng Physick (1815) of Philadelphia developed an ingenious dilatation system with metal catheters and animal skin balloons (Shelly 1969).

The first prostatectomy to be carried out in Britain was performed in the Leeds General Infirmary by Arthur Fergusson McGill in 1887. At the annual meeting of the British Medical Association held in Leeds in 1889 McGill led the discussion on the treatment of retention of urine due to prostatic enlargement. He put forward a number of interesting points for discussion: that patients who can catheterise without discomfort do not need surgery; that when catheterisation fails, radical surgery is essential; that such radical treatment needs to achieve free drainage of the bladder and

asthma and diabetes are all within the remit of internal medicine, rather than surgically based as is the case with BPH, so there has been little resistance from family practitioners to taking on gradually the extra burden of management of these conditions. In an interesting parallel with prostatic disease, hypertension is generally considered to be appropriately managed at the family practitioner level; angina, by contrast, is usually regarded as an indication for specialist referral – presumably because of the invasive testing and therapy by angiography and angioplasty, as well as the unpredictable risk of sudden death from myocardial infarction. Similarly, it seems likely that whereas uncomplicated, mild-to-moderate BPH may become the province of the family practitioner, prostate cancer (or suspicions thereof) will always prompt referral for evaluation by a urologist.

The shared care initiative for BPH

In order to harmonise thoughts on these matters a committee was formed in 1994 under the chairmanship of the late Professor Geoffrey Chisholm CBE. The issues surrounding the presentation, evaluation and guidelines for referral were discussed and a nomogram devised (Kirby *et al.* 1995) (see Figure 2.1). The feasibility and overall acceptance of the precepts and assumptions contained within that nomogram were field-tested by means of a questionnaire sent to 2,020 urologists, general surgeons with an interest in urology, geriatricians, family health service advisers and general practitioners. The absolute numbers and percentage of responders for each group are shown in Table 2.1.

Results of the survey

There was consensus that screening for BPH (i.e. inviting men aged between 50 and 70 years to attend for a prostate health check) was not generally practicable, although pilot screening studies in the UK have confirmed a 2 per cent pick-up rate of apparently significant prostate cancer (Kirby *et al.* 1994). By contrast, the prospect of *case*

Table 2.1 Responders to the questionnaire sent out by the Shared Care Initiative Committee

Group	No. sent	Response	
		No.	*%*
Urologists	320	159	49.7
General surgeons	373	85	22.8
Geriatricians	712	160	22.5
Family practitioners	500	118	23.6
FHSA advisers	115	58	50.4
Total	2,020	580	28.7

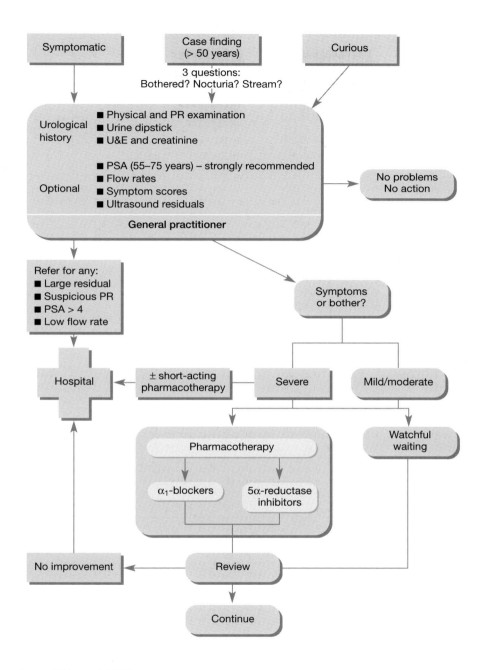

Source: Kirby *et al.* (1995)

Figure 2.1 Managing clinical BPH: the shared care initiative

finding was greeted with more enthusiasm. In this setting the American Urological Association (AUA) symptom scores or International Prostate Symptom Score (IPSS) with their seven questions and possible cumulative score of 35 were regarded as too cumbersome. Instead, it was proposed that the family practitioner could readily ask all male patients of more than 50 years of age, presenting for whatever reason, the following key questions:

- do you get up at night to pass urine?
- is your urinary stream reduced?
- are you 'bothered' by your bladder function?

Individuals responding positively to any of these questions might then be administered a targeted AUA/IPSS symptom score and undergo a physical examination.

Physical examination for the symptomatic patient in whom BPH is suspected should include a focused neurological examination, as well as a palpation of the lower abdomen to exclude a chronically distended bladder. The cornerstone of the physical assessment is the digital rectal examination (DRE). Most respondents agreed that DRE was mandatory in the evaluation of BPH patients and that any induration or palpable nodule present should be regarded as an indication for referral to a urologist to exclude a diagnosis of prostate cancer. More work is necessary, however, to educate family practitioners in the skills of DRE, as a survey in the UK suggested that the majority were performing less than five of these examinations per month (Hennigan *et al.* 1990).

The issue of prostate cancer raises the question of the necessity for PSA testing. Respondents to the questionnaire were almost equally divided in their opinions. Although PSA testing will undoubtedly diagnose cases of early prostate cancer, there was concern that many patients, especially those in the mildly elevated PSA ranges, would be unnecessarily alarmed, perhaps undergo transrectal ultrasound-guided biopsy and, in fact, be found to have BPH. For this reason, PSA was included as an optional (but recommended) test for men aged between 50 and 70 years with prostatic symptoms, rather than a formal guideline requirement. The American Healthcare Policy Review (AHCPR) guideline committee came to similar conclusions (McConnell *et al.* 1994).

Who to refer?

The respondents generally agreed with the following guidelines for recommended patient referral to a urologist:

- severe symptoms (IPSS >18)
- history of haematuria
- palpably distended bladder or chronic retention on ultrasound

- abnormal DRE (especially a palpable nodule or prostatic induration)
- raised serum creatinine
- raised PSA (>4 ng/ml)
- any patient about whose diagnosis or treatment the GP has concern.

Who to treat?

It is now legitimate for family practitioners to start medical therapy in uncomplicated BPH, either with an α-blocker or a 5α-reductase inhibitor. Those patients with mild symptoms (IPSS <8) and who have little 'bother' from their BPH will usually be more appropriately managed by watchful waiting and annual review.

Follow-up for those managed medically

Patients with moderate symptoms of BPH and a normal DRE, normal PSA and creatinine values and who are managed medically will need to be reviewed regularly to monitor treatment response and evaluate side-effects. The frequency of these follow-up visits will depend on the particular agent selected for therapy.

Which drug therapy?

In general, α-blockers have a rapid onset of action in terms of symptom alleviation and flow rate improvement (Eri & Tveter 1995), but most require careful dose titration to minimise side-effects of dizziness and postural hypotension. Doxazosin and terazosin, for example, should be started at 1 mg/day and gradually increased to a maintenance dosage of 4 or 5 mg/day, respectively (some patients may benefit from a further dose increment to 8 or 10 mg, respectively). Patients treated thus should be reviewed in a timely fashion for these dose adjustments. Longer-term follow-up is also necessary because although α-blockers relieve symptoms and improve peak flow rates, they do not reverse the underlying pathophysiology and prostate growth is likely to continue.

5α-reductase inhibitors, such as finasteride, have a slower onset of action but achieve, eventually, a level of symptom reduction and peak flow rate enhancement which is beneficial to a proportion of patients (Gormley *et al.* 1992; Stoner & the Finasteride Study Group 1994), particularly when prostate size is greater than 40 cc (Boyle *et al.* 1996). Moreover, as they shrink the prostate and reverse the underlying pathophysiology of BPH, they may prevent longer-term complications, such as acute retention, and reduce the need for eventual surgery (Andersen *et al.* 1995; McConnell *et al.* 1998). Finasteride also suppresses serum PSA levels (because PSA secretion is an androgen-dependent process) to around 50 per cent of pre-treatment values within 6–12 months of therapy (Gaches *et al.* 1979). Patients treated medically for BPH should ideally be reviewed at three-month intervals. Failure of PSA reduction and, in particular, evidence of an increase in PSA in spite of finasteride therapy, or failure to control symptoms, should prompt referral to a urologist for the exclusion of an occult prostate cancer.

Potential benefits of shared care

The algorithm featured in Figure 2.1 provides a framework for urologists and family practitioners to work together to optimise therapy for the many millions of sufferers from this most prevalent disease. Although some will argue that each patient with symptomatic BPH should, ideally, be seen and evaluated by a urologist, logistics alone suggest that this will not be possible. In the UK there are an estimated 2.5 million men with symptomatic BPH but only approximately 430 urologists; by contrast, there are around 33,000 family practitioners.

In order for shared care of BPH to work effectively there are learning steps to be climbed by family practitioners. These are depicted in Figure 2.2. Urologists will need to involve themselves in this process of educating their colleagues in primary care in such skills as DRE and PSA interpretation.

Shared care for BPH in practice should permit more rapid access for patients to appropriate investigation and treatment. Family practitioners should benefit by being able to offer a more comprehensive range of therapies for their patients, as they gain experience in the management of BPH. Urologists should also gain, by building bridges between themselves and the family practitioners who refer to them. This will

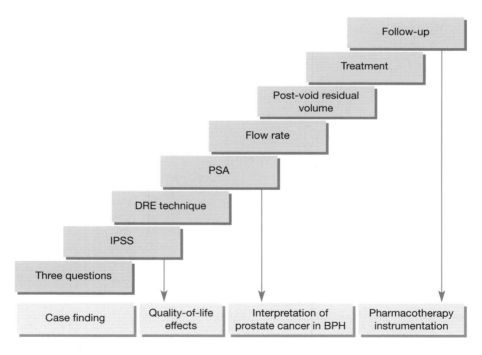

Figure 2.2 Education of family practitioners by urologists: the learning steps

ensure that they see an increasing number of properly selected and carefully assessed patients who particularly require their special operative and interventional skills.

Shared care in the real world: a review of the experience of one unit

In early 1992 we (AB and TMcN) developed a nurse practitioner-run clinic for the rapid assessment of men with LUTS in North Hertfordshire. Seven years later, we are in a position to discuss the concept of nurse-run assessment clinics with a great deal more experience and to form a view as to whether these developments have been helpful in improving access to the various treatment options for BPH and have facilitated sharing the care of men with LUTS with our GP colleagues.

During this period there has been an upheaval in British health care, with the formal separation of providers from purchasers and the introduction of the internal market, and the demand for urological specialists has increased dramatically. The underlying reason driving our initiative was the need to develop a means of offering fast and efficient assessment of men with BPH to the large symptomatic population. This could not be managed by the existing urological specialists and led to the recruitment of trained urological specialist nurses (USN) in several urological departments or in community units providing non-specialist care for 'continence' services to the general population.

This development was designed as an alternative to the traditional model involving patient referral to a specialist in secondary care. Our aim was to improve the management of men with LUTS in the general population, especially where urological specialist services were limited, and thus avoid delay in symptomatic men receiving help. In particular, we hoped to improve access to the basic measurements so that each patient would have the opportunity to be considered for medical treatment. In addition, we hoped to generate greater awareness among family or general practitioners of what could and should be measured and how to use these parameters in combination with their own personal knowledge of a patient's circumstances.

We encouraged two (and later three) experienced urological nurses who provided community continence services locally to focus on the assessment of men with LUTS. They had secretarial assistance, an office, telephones and three (then four) community-based clinic sites in which to assess men with a range of flowmeters and bladder ultrasound scanners. They were trained in venepuncture and became familiar with administering and assessing symptom scores. They were already expert at dealing with urine specimens for microbiological and cytological examination and they followed a protocol that was agreed between the specialist urologists and local GPs (Figure 2.2, opposite) and which is broadly similar to many national protocols that were published in the UK subsequently.

GPs could refer individual patients to the USN clinic for assessment. These were then seen by the clinic within one month, which compared favourably with the existing waiting time for a specialist clinic appointment. Charges were set at a level approximately half that of the specialist clinic. The aim was to perform as similar an assessment as possible to the 'traditional' urological clinic work-up for men with LUTS (see Figures 2.3 and 2.4). This, it was hoped, would allow identification of a group of men requiring specialist attention. GPs could then watch or medically treat others as appropriate, and could have their patients reassessed by the specialist nurses when there was a need to measure response to any treatment or to see if deterioration was occurring (particularly for those on watchful waiting). The nurses

---

❏ Introduction of patient to the assessment

❏ Dietary enquiry

❏ Voiding diaries (previously sent to patient if possible)

❏ Administer symptom scores (IPSS)

❏ Flowmetry (maximum urinary flow (Qmax), average flow, voiding volume)

❏ Transabdominal ultrasound bladder scan (measures residual urine)

❏ Digital rectal examination (DRE) – introduced later after training

❏ Venepuncture (for PSA, creatinine, urea and electrolytes)

❏ Urinalysis (SG10 'stix' to detect blood, protein, leucocyte esterase and nitrite)

❏ Cytology (particularly if predominantly 'irritable' bladder symptoms)

Figure 2.3 Nurse assessment in clinic

❏ Severe symptoms

❏ Haematuria

❏ Renal impairment

❏ Recurrent UTIs

❏ Palpable bladder
  – acute retention
  – chronic retention
  – residual urine +200 ml

❏ Raised PSA >4
  (PSA 4–10 depends on patient age, DRE and GP's opinion)

Figure 2.4 Nurse assessment: standard indications for referral

1	Referred to specialist clinic
2	Watchful waiting – bladder retraining protocols – altering fluid intake and drinking habits
3	Medical therapy – α-blocker therapy – α-reductase inhibitor (finasteride)

Figure 2.5 Nurse assessment: outcomes

had the opportunity to advise on simple methods of dealing with LUTS by bladder-retraining protocols and by altering fluid intake and drinking habits (Figure 2.5). A multi-part report form was designed and top copies of the assessment were sent to GPs; one copy was also given directly to the patient and one was stored for audit and future reference.

During the period October 1992–September 1998, 1,259 men passed through the community-based assessment and treatment clinic. The first 50 were part of a pilot study during which the protocol and mechanisms were being refined. There was a steady decrease in the numbers being referred on for specialist urological assessment and management (Table 2.2).

Overall, 55 per cent of men were managed entirely in the community by their GPs without specialist referral. Generally, there was a growing trend towards less specialist referral as GPs became more familiar with the concepts involved and more experienced in the management of BPH. In 1998 this trend altered slightly with an increase of 4 per cent in referrals to urological specialists. This is thought to be due to an increase in men failing medical treatment. GPs may also have been referring more complex cases to the nurse clinics, larger proportions of whom might then have needed referral.

Table 2.2 Eventual site of management of 1,259 men reviewed in the North Herts community-based assessment clinic (1992–8)

	Community Management (GP/nurses) (%)	Urological Management (Specialist) (%)
Overall 1992–8	55	45
1993	41	59
1994	51	49
1995	59	41
1998	54	45

An audit of the community-based assessment clinic was performed (funded by a grant from Abbott Pharmaceuticals, UK). Table 2.3 shows the overall outcome of 690 men reviewed by September 1995 and the results of two sub-groups that were looked at in more detail in that year. These are discussed below.

Of the 310 men referred for specialist urological assessment by September 1995, approximately 20 per cent (70 men) were looked at in greater detail and all their studies were repeated in the specialist clinic. In all 70 men the two assessments substantially agreed; there was one minor difference that was not clinically significant. This strongly suggested that the measurements made in the community were as sensitive and reliable as those being made in the specialist clinic.

The main reasons for referral from the rapid-access community clinic were reviewed. A raised PSA (>4) was the single most important reason (30 per cent). High symptom scores led to referral in 21 per cent and low flow rates to a further 21 per cent, though most patients had several indications for referral. Of the men seen by the specialists, further investigations were required in 16 (usually transrectal ultrasound examination and/or pressure flow cystometry). Thirty-six underwent surgical treatment, 21 medical treatment and in 11 watchful waiting was chosen. Two men were treated for prostate cancer.

Table 2.3 The community-based assessment and treatment of BPH
(Oct 1992–Sept 1995) (n= 690 men)

310 (45%)	Referred to urological department
70 (19%)	Studies repeated
	69 of 70 agreed
	1 minor difference
Further investigations 16	(TRUS in 10; urodynamics in 6)
Management	
Surgical	36
Medical	21
Watchful waiting	11
Hormonal	2 (Cancer of the prostate)
380 (55%)	Offered 'non-surgical' management
75 (19.7%)	Offered specialist review + DRE at 18.5 months later (range 4–43 months)
54 (72%)	Attended
	general agreement (Biochem N/A)
	5 men at significant risk of cancer of the prostate
	4 on DRE, 1 on PSA
	(abnormal at first visit)

However, in many ways the most interesting group of patients from this cohort were those who were *not* being referred to a specialist urologist, and we attempted to review a representative sub-group of the 380 men who had been managed entirely in the community by their GPs following assessment by the USN. Approximately 20 per cent of these (75 men) were offered a second review in the same community clinic and by the same staff, but with the addition of a specialist urologist who reviewed the patients and performed a DRE. Of the 75 men, 54 agreed to attend (72 per cent) and again there was general agreement between the first and second assessment, despite the mean of 18.5 months (range 4–43 months) between the two assessments. However, one clear deficiency in the previous assessment showed up: five men (9.3 per cent) were thought to be at significant risk of having prostatic cancer on the second assessment, four on the basis of an abnormal DRE and one on the basis of an abnormal PSA (which had been abnormal at his first visit and had therefore been missed due to an administrative error).

Details of the characteristics of patients at first and second consultation are shown in Table 2.4, from which it can be seen that approximately 7.4 per cent of men in a group with otherwise reassuring features were felt to have an abnormal DRE suggestive of prostate cancer.

There was a reduction in men with predominantly irritable bladder symptoms, presumably due to the bladder retraining offered at the clinic. There was a small increase in the percentage with evidence of infection (3.7 per cent from 1.5 per cent). Overall, approximately 60 per cent in both groups were treated by a combination

Table 2.4 Results of first and second consultations (mean follow-up period 18.5 months between consultations)

	Consultation 1	*Consultation 2*
Age	33–83	35–83
Urinalysis	4% msu+ve	8%+ve
DRE done	19 (35%)	54 (100%)
DRE abnormal	0*	4 (7.4%)
Diagnosis		
Freq/urg	59%	48%
BOO/BPH	35%	33%
UTI /prostatitis	1.5%	3.7%
Possible prostate cancer	0%	9.3%
Treatment		
Watchful waiting/retraining	60%	57%
Medical	30%	30%
Referral	0%	9.3% (4+1)

* GPs were asked to refer men if DRE was abnormal

of watchful waiting, bladder retraining and advice about fluid intake. Thirty per cent of men at both assessments were put on medical treatment and approximately 10 per cent of this cohort should have been referred for specialist urological management on the basis of the suspicion of prostate cancer found at the second consultation.

The most significant feature of this study is that only 35 per cent of the men reviewed either remembered having a DRE by their GP or had written evidence of that examination. While this may greatly underestimate the number of patients who really had a DRE, it does suggest a weakness in the system in the UK where DREs are infrequently performed and GPs often volunteer that they are inadequately trained and inexperienced in digitally examining the prostate (Hennigan *et al.* 1990).

Conclusions

As a result of these findings we conclude that interested GPs and trained USNs could safely identify men with LUTS not requiring immediate specialist care, who could be safely observed or treated medically in the community if more attention was paid to DRE. More training in DRE is needed, although the importance of diagnosing prostate cancer will depend on national attitudes to the detection and treatment of (early) disease. Such attitudes vary widely both internationally and within the UK.

There may be an expanding role for USNs, here, in providing a supply of health care professionals trained, assessed and experienced in DRE, particularly where primary medical services are stretched to the limit, as in the UK. Our nurses themselves are keen and have been restrained until recently by our uncertainties about just what is expected of them: are they to perform a purely 'prostatic' examination, or is it a pelvic or ano-rectal examination? Each extention of the process would obviously require more complex training, and medico-legal issues would also need to be tackled.

For both the patient and the specialist there have been obvious advantages: patients are referred with most of the essential information a specialist needs, so that a decision on treatment can often be made at their first specialist consultation. There are clear benefits for the GP too. Taking into account time pressures and other existing responsibilities, such as the management of diabetes, hypertension or asthma, which are well established in UK general practice, this model offers the GP the flexibility of being involved in the management of BPH to the degree they desire and with the easily accessible means of categorising men into groups suitable for management by GP or who require referral to a specialist.

Benign prostatic hyperplasia – quality of life patient survey

The North Hertfordshire assessment service receives referrals from 26 local GP practices. Over 550 men assessed at the clinic have been diagnosed as suffering from BPH. The majority of these patients were treated by one of the following three treatment modalities: medical management, surgery or watchful waiting.

A patient survey in 1998 was designed to review the impact of these treatment modalities upon quality of life and the progression of the disease. Results from the survey (Table 2.5) highlight the significant role that medical management plays in the treatment of BPH, with nearly six out of every ten men who replied initially being treated with the 5α-reductase inhibitor, finasteride, or an α-blocker. Of those who received medical management, one third were prescribed finasteride and 60 per cent received an α-blocker.

Clinical evidence suggests that finasteride is mostly beneficial to those men with enlarged prostates, i.e. >40 cc (Boyle *et al.* 1996). Epidemiological studies suggest that approximately 20 per cent of men aged 70–79 years have this degree of prostatic enlargement (Garraway *et al.* 1991). Given the fact that men presenting to their physician are self-selecting, the actual percentage of men with enlarged prostates will be greater. Consequently, the distribution of medical therapies initiated at the prostate disease assessment service would suggest an appropriate distribution of therapy use. However, clinical records must be investigated to clarify whether prescribing is being appropriately tailored to individual patients.

The reported median 'bother' and symptom scores for the two therapies are statistically equivalent, although the 'bother' score for finasteride was slightly better than that reported for α-blockers. The median scores for 'bother' and symptoms reported were lower in the medical treatment groups than the watchful waiting group, although this was not statistically significant.

It may be assumed that the level reported by the watchful waiting group reflects the threshold of symptoms and 'bother' that patients are willing to accept. Consequently, these results show that medical management is associated with a level of symptoms and 'bother' that patients find acceptable to live with. The survey does not allow the degree of reduction in symptoms and bother levels associated with different interventions to be evaluated.

Nearly six in ten of these patients who initially received medical treatment remained on this therapy (Figure 2.6), with three-quarters having done so for over one year. This implied degree of compliance suggests that medical treatment is conferring clinically important benefits to these patients.

Table 2.5 Survey of men attending N Herts prostate disease assessment service (n=257)

Treatment option chosen	No.	(%)
Tablet	147	57.2
Bladder retraining	4	1.6
Surgery	27	10.5
Watchful waiting	28	10.9
Other	8	3.1
None	36	14.0
Missing	7	2.7

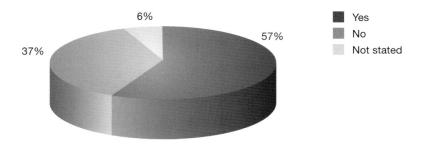

6%

37%

57%

■ Yes
■ No
 Not stated

Figure 2.6 Number of men still taking tablets for their prostate problem (n=147)

Nearly one in ten patients who returned the questionnaire went on to develop acute urinary retention (AUR), with no significant difference between the medical therapy and watchful waiting groups. However, no patients treated with finasteride developed AUR compared to 9 per cent of patients treated with an α-blocker. Although not statistically significant, these data reflect findings from PLESS (Proscar Long-term Efficacy and Safety Study) showing that finasteride significantly reduces the risk of AUR (McConnell *et al.* 1998).

Forty men required surgery after first visiting the prostate disease assessment service. It is interesting to note that of these, nearly two-thirds had already undergone a surgical procedure for the disease. However, these patients reported a significantly lower median symptom and 'bother' score than those in the watchful waiting or medical management groups.

One in ten of the men who underwent surgery were not at all satisfied with the outcome (Figure 2.7) and were more likely to have experienced surgical complications such as bleeding requiring a transfusion, incontinence and ejaculation problems. This reflects the 10–20 per cent of patients who are reported in the National Prostatectomy Audit to be less than completely satisfied with their treatment (Emberton *et al.* 1995). It has been estimated that outcomes could be improved in those dissatisfied by means of better case selection and, where necessary, formal urodynamic evaluation in up to 50 per cent of cases (Speakman *et al.* 1987).

Only one third (33 per cent) of the men included in the study had been sexually active in the last month. These men on average were fairly satisfied with their level of sexual activity.

In terms of follow-up and review of patients, significantly more patients (three out of four men) who had had surgery were not followed up by a health care professional, compared to those who received medical treatment or were managed by watchful waiting (Figure 2.8). More than half those patients treated by the latter two modalities said that they were reviewed less than once a year.

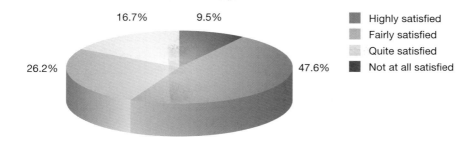

Figure 2.7 Level of satisfaction with surgery (n=42)

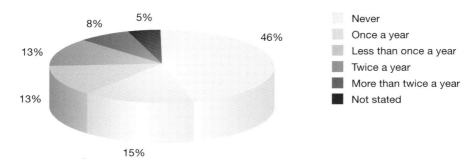

Figure 2.8 Frequency of follow-up after treatment (n=257)

The interpretation of these data may be prone to bias, in that it is likely that those patients with moderate or severe symptoms/bother were more motivated to return the questionnaire. While the survey provides some interesting insights into the management of BPH and its impact upon patients, these data must be reviewed in the light of their relatively subjective nature.

Conclusions

The situation and responses described above are specifically relevant to the UK and may not be relevant elsewhere. The traditional model of a medical specialist assessment is an excellent option if resources allow. However, in the UK it has been found that the current provision for the management of LUTS cannot cope without prolonged waiting and rationing of urological expertise. The shared care model described offers one means of improving access for symptomatic men to safe and effective assessment, advice and treatment. It only works if the assessment is still sufficiently skilled and accurate. The assessment should include measurement of the severity and bother of symptoms, the degree of obstruction, the presence or absence of absolute indicators of the need for specialist referral and the size of the prostate. There is a role for the careful observation of the condition if not severe (i.e. 'watchful waiting') and medical therapies are now established as reasonable treatment options for the more bothered. Both do require periodic review to allow change of the treatment plan if circumstances alter. New treatment technologies may play an increasingly important role but are currently still largely investigational and seem to require more complex assessment and therefore referral to a specialist urological service.

References

Andersen JT, Ekman P, Wolf M *et al.* (1995). Can finasteride reverse the progress of benign prostatic hyperplasia? A two-year placebo-controlled study. *Urology* **46**, 631–7.

Ashton Miller J & Staunton MD (1989). The birth of retropubic prostatectomy – Millin. *J Roy Soc Med* **82**, 494–5.

Boyle P, Gould A & Roehrborn C (1996). Prostate volume predicts outcome of treatment of benign prostatic hyperplasia with finasteride: meta-analysis of randomized clinical trials. *Urology* **48**, 398–405.

Caine M, Pfau A & Perlberg S (1976). The use of alpha-adrenergic blockers in benign prostatic obstruction. *Br J Urol* **48**, 255–63.

Clark P (1987). Centenary of the first prostatectomy in Britain. *Br J Urol* **60**, 549–53.

Denis L, McConnell J, Yoshida O *et al.* (1997). Recommendations of the international scientific committee: the evaluation and treatment of lower urinary tract symptoms (LUTS) suggestive of benign prostatic obstruction. In *4th International Consultation on Benign Prostatic Hyperplasia (BPH)* vol.4 (ed. L Denis, K Griffiths, S Khoury), pp. 669–84. SCI, Paris.

Emberton M, Neal D, Black N *et al.* (1995). The national prostatectomy audit: the clinical management of patients during hospital admission. *B J Urol* **75**, 301–16.

Eri LM & Tveter KJ (1995). Alpha-blockade in the treatment of symptomatic benign prostatic hyperplasia. *J Urol* **154**, 923–34.

Freyer P (1900). A new method of performing prostatectomy. *Lancet* **1**, 774–5.

Gaches C, Asken M, Dunn M & Hammonds J (1979). The role of selective internal urethrotomy in the management of urethral strictures: a multi-centre education. *B J Urol* **51**, 579–83.

Garraway W, Collins G & Lee R (1991). High prevalence of benign prostatic hypertrophy in the community. *Lancet* **338**, 469–71.

Gormley GJ, Stoner E, Bruskewitz RC *et al.* (1992). The effect of finasteride in men with benign prostatic hyperplasia. *N E J M* **327**, 1185–91.

Hennigan TW, Franks PJ, Hocken DB & Allen-Mersh TG (1990). Rectal examination in general practice. *BMJ* **301**, 478–80.

Kirby RS, Kirby MG, Feneley MR, McNicholas T, McLean A & Webb J (1994). Screening for carcinoma of the prostate: a GP based study. *Br J Urol* **74**, 64–71.

Kirby RS, Chisholm G, Chapple CR *et al.* (1995). Shared care between general practitioners and urologists in the management of benign prostatic hyperplasia: a survey of attitudes among clinicians. *J R Soc Med* **88**, 284–8.

Lepor H, Willaford W, Barry M, Brawer M, Dickson C & Gormley G (1996). The efficacy of terazosin, finasteride or both in benign prostatic hyperplasia. Veteran's Affairs Co-operative Studies Benign Prostatic Hyperplasia Study Group. *N E J M* **335**, 533–9.

McCarthy J (1931). A new apparatus for endoscopic plastic surgery of the prostate. *J Urol* **26**, 695–6.

McConnell JD, Barry MJ, Bruskewitz RC *et al.* (1994). *Benign prostatic hyperplasia: diagnosis and treatment.* Clinical Practice Guideline No. 8, pp. 1–225. US Department of Health and Human Resources, Rockville (Md), USA.

McConnell J, Bruskewitz R, Walsh P *et al.* (1998). The effect of finasteride on the risk of acute urinary retention and the need for surgical treatment among men with benign prostatic hyperplasia. *N E J M* **338**(9), 557–63.

Orton P (1994). Shared care. *Lancet* **344**, 1413–15.

Shelly H (1969). The enlarged prostate. A brief history of its treatment. *J Hist Med* **Oct**, 452–73.

Speakman M, Sethia K, Fellows G & Smith J (1987). A study of the pathogenesis, urodynamic assessment and outcome of detrusor instability associated with bladder outflow obstruction. *B J Urol* **59**, 40–4.

Stoner E and the Finasteride Study Group (1992). The clinical effects of 5 alpha reductase inhibitor, Finasteride, on benign prostatic hyperplasia. *J Urol* **147**, 1298–302.

Stoner E and the Finasteride Study Group (1994). Three-year safety and efficacy data on the use of finasteride in the treatment of benign prostatic hyperplasia. *Urology* **43**, 284–94.

Chapter 3

Specialist investigations for the man with lower urinary tract symptoms

Simon St Clair Carter

Introduction

One of the main problems in the field of urology is defining what we understand by a 'patient with BPH'. To the scientist, the term conveys a man with a particular histological diagnosis; to the educated health care professional, a physiological problem of obstruction; and to most patients, a set of symptoms commonly associated with ageing. For the modern urologist, the definition is a combination of all three, as shown in the famous diagram of Ter Hald (1989). He has used a Venn diagram or set to describe the conventional patient with lower urinary tract symptoms (LUTS), benign prostatic enlargement (BPE) and bladder outflow obstruction (BOO) (Figure 3.1). However, anybody involved in recruiting patients for clinical trials of treatments of BPH will know how frustratingly few men seen in their daily clinics fall exactly into this central domain.

Men need assessment of their prostate and lower urinary tract for a number of reasons. Usually, we assess patients because they have some symptoms, even though in some these may not be causing them any significant impact on their well-being.

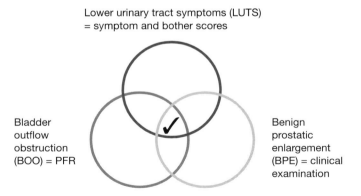

Figure 3.1 The three rings of Hald describing the factors involved in the definition of the BPH patient with the simple tests used to define each category. The tick marks the domain of the traditional patient with all three factors present

Increasingly, we see people who wish to be screened for prostatic cancer or want to be certain that their benign disease will not deteriorate, if left untreated, or result in complications in the future. We are also called upon to investigate the patient who has been told by another health care worker that there is a problem, perhaps that the prostate is large or that there is a large residual urine in the absence of symptoms.

The real importance of BPH for the urologist is in treating and avoiding the complications of BOO. Most result from changes in bladder function, such as retention, overactivity or recurrent infection due to an increased residual volume (Comiter *et al.* 1997). It would seem therefore to be sensible to modify the Venn diagram of Ter Hald to include a fourth category for bladder function (Figure 3.2). Such a set has 15 possible domains (see Table 3.1), and each ideally should have a clinical management strategy clearly defined. Although this might appear complex, it is in fact often the state of the bladder that prompts us to advise one treatment over another (Jensen *et al.* 1988; Blaivas 1996). This chapter describes how a patient can be allocated to each of these domains.

Classification of patients is either achieved by the use of less precise, but simple non-invasive investigations, or more precise, more complex, often invasive, specialist tests. Symptom assessment, including measurement of the impact on the patient's quality of life, should be the starting point (Roehrborn *et al.* 1995). However, some symptoms in men with a suspicion of BPH may require clarification with a variety of other urological investigations, including cystoscopy, detailed microbiological survey and assessment of the fluid balance status. The definitive investigation for the assessment of obstruction and bladder function is the voiding cystometrogram and, for the definition of prostatic anatomy, a transrectal ultrasound study (Aarnink *et al.* 1998). Table 3.2 lists the investigations under consideration.

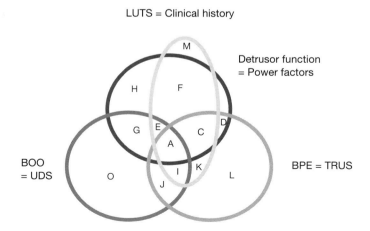

Figure 3.2 A modification of Hald's rings to include abnormalities of bladder function and the more complex tests used to describe each category

Table 3.1 The 15 possible domains of the modified description of lower urinary tract function, as shown in Figure 3.2

Category	LUTS	BPH	Bladder outflow obstruction	Detrusor failure
A	✓	✓	✓	✓
B	✓	✓	✓	–
C	✓	✓	–	✓
D	✓	✓	–	–
E	✓	–	✓	✓
F	✓	–	–	✓
G	✓	–	✓	–
H	✓	–	–	–
I	–	✓	✓	✓
J	–	✓	✓	–
K	–	✓	–	✓
L	–	✓	–	–
N	–	–	✓	✓
M	–	–	–	✓
O	–	–	✓	–

Table 3.2 Investigations required to classify the pathophysiology of a man with benign prostatic disease

Characteristic	Investigations	
	Simple	Complex
Benign prostatic enlargement (BPE)	Digital rectal examination (DRE)	Transrectal ultrasound (TRUS)
Lower urinary tract symptoms (LUTS)	Symptom score Bother score	Frequency–volume chart (FV chart)
Bladder outflow obstruction (BOO)	Peak flow rate (PFR)	Pressure flow study (PFS)
Detrusor function	Post-void residual (PVR)	Full urodynamic study (UDS)
Lower urinary tract symptoms (LUTS)	Symptom score Bother score	Frequency–volume chart Cystoscopy Microbiological survey

Why undertake complex assessment?

In an ideal world, any patient seeking help would be advised as to the best treatment on the basis of a scientifically precise diagnosis. In clinical practice we often have to rely on imprecise diagnosis and administer treatments in the expectation that the outcome in the majority of patients will be satisfactory. Nowhere is this truer than in the treatment of the man with LUTS, as the precise definition of the pathophysiological problem can only be achieved by complex and invasive investigation. We rely on simple, less accurate investigations in the first instance in order to avoid distress, discomfort and morbidity from the process of investigation. Patients who fall into Ter Hald's central area domain (A) (see Figure 3.2, on p.40), as defined by systematic symptom assessment, digital examination and flow rate, fit the entry criteria for many of the therapeutic clinical trials, and the response to treatment can be predicted with some certainty. For most such patients who find the symptoms bothersome a trial of medical treatment, such as an alpha-blocking agent, is advised, and complex assessment would seem to be inappropriate (McConnell *et al.* 1994). If medical therapy fails, some form of excisional surgery, such as transurethral resection of the prostate (TURP), is usually advised and again the outcome in the traditional patient from the central area domain is well known and satisfactory in about 85 per cent (Neal *et al.* 1989).

The most cogent argument for the precise definition of the pathophysiological problem in any given patient is that it would allow better selection between different treatment modalities (Steers & Zorn 1995; Jepsen & Bruskewitz 1998). In earlier times the urological community used the rather hopeful approach that a single modality of treatment (TURP) might be effective in dealing with all men with symptoms suggestive of BPH. With experience the criteria were redefined: patients with normal flow rates were excluded and fewer patients were submitted to surgery. However, even today, a TURP is recommended to patients on the basis of symptoms and a low flow rate without consideration of the prostate size when more simple procedures such as bladder neck incision or transurethral incision of the prostate might be more suitable methods of decreasing outflow resistance. The advent of effective pharmacological therapy in the form of safe alpha-blocking agents and 5α reductase inhibitors has led once more to less precise selection for treatment, in that any patient with symptoms is likely to be offered drug therapy before being comprehensively assessed by flow rates and ultrasound examination (Abrams 1995). Information to show that effectiveness can be improved by case selection has been slow in coming but will probably accumulate rapidly in the future. Already, there is powerful evidence to suggest that the use of finasteride in patients with large prostates is more effective than in those with smaller glands (Boyle *et al.* 1996). Some would now argue that it is inappropriate to subject patients to surgical intervention without having a definitive physiological and anatomical assessment (Thomas & Abrams 1998). Although evidence to support an improved outcome from more detailed pre-operative assessment remains difficult to find, the prevailing climate of criticism of poor surgical results will inevitably lead to the use of more complex definitive investigations.

One of the spurs to the more widespread use of complex investigations has been the development of alternative technological therapies to treat prostatic obstruction. The various novel treatments may not be suitable for all sizes or shapes of prostate. As an example, the use of low-energy transurethral microwave therapy (TUMT) with a hot point below the bladder neck has been shown to be more effective in patients with prostatic obstruction than bladder neck obstruction, and high-energy TUMT is known to be more effective in larger and more obstructive prostates (Tubaro *et al.* 1995; de-Wildt *et al.* 1996). It is likely that, as new treatments become more mature, more complex investigations will be needed in order to identify the ideal patient for each therapy. A systematic plan of investigation should be employed in all patients before treatment is recommended and particularly before using newer treatments of lesser efficacy and of often uncertain durability.

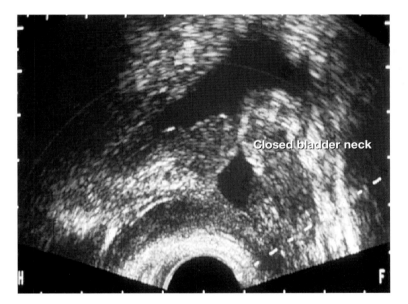

Figure 3.3 The sagittal transrectal ultrasound image of a patient treated with a low-energy programme with the hot point 10 mm below the bladder neck. Despite obliteration of the prostatic lateral lobes, the bladder neck remains intact and urodynamics show obstruction

Which patients should be selected for complex assessment?

At present patients are selected for more complex investigation on the basis of the history, clinical examination or the results of first-line investigations (see Table 3.3) (Chapple 1993). Conventional problems of diagnosis arise in patients where the symptoms are not typical of simple BPH. Symptoms which may merit further

Table 3.3 Patients who should be selected for complex assessment

- Men with atypical symptoms such as:
  - pain
  - urgency
  - incontinence

- Patients with other diseases affecting lower urinary tract:
  - neurological disease
  - diabetes
  - abnormalities of urine production

- Post-surgical or interventional treatment failures

- Symptomatic patients with any of the following:
  - small prostates
  - normal flow rates
  - large residual urine

- Men without LUTS but who have an incidental finding of:
  - a large residual urine
  - a very large prostate

- Those wishing to avoid retrograde ejaculation

- High-risk patients (e.g. cardiopaths and anticoagulated)

- For reasons of cost containment

consideration include pain suggestive of prostatitis, excessive urgency of micturition and incontinence. Patients with these symptoms often have other diseases (e.g. urinary or genital tract infection, abnormal renal function, neurological problems and diabetes), which may have an impact on lower urinary tract function. Perhaps the most difficult group of men requiring complex investigation are those in whom previous interventional and surgical procedures have failed to produce a satisfactory outcome or have resulted in significant complications. These patients are increasing in number because of the use of multiple experimental treatments leading to partially successful outcomes.

The most common reason for further investigation is when, despite a clinical picture of BOO causing LUTS, the initial simple tests do not confirm the diagnosis. Typically, this would be a man with a small prostate and normal urinary flow rates; however, also patients with a large prostate and a normal flow, or a low flow and a small prostate, should also be considered for further study. It is increasingly common to see a patient without specific urinary symptoms but in whom an ultrasound examination has revealed significant residual urine or a large prostate. Such findings may be discovered because the patient was assessed for early prostate cancer in a prostate assessment clinic. While his anxieties regarding prostate cancer may have been relieved, he has been informed of a new possible cause of disease and naturally wishes to be reassured that there will be no significant adverse impact on his future health.

Patients with co-morbidity such as severe cardiac or respiratory disease and those on long-term anticoagulation therapy may need a more detailed assessment of the problem because the risks of surgery are greater for them. Younger patients with symptoms which are sufficiently severe to require an interventional or surgical treatment that might produce changes in sexual and reproductive function may wish to be certain that the procedure will be of benefit before agreeing to treatment.

The important issues of cost containment may also be an indication for the complex investigation of patients. We have shown before that the routine use of urodynamic studies before performing a TURP is economic if patients without obstruction, as defined by pressure flow studies, or with equivocal obstruction are treated by other means, including watchful waiting, pharmacological therapy or minimally invasive therapies (Walker *et al.* 1997a). Such arguments can only be valid if the patients can be effectively treated by other means and that the outcome of surgery is shown to be less likely to be successful in the absence of urodynamically defined obstruction. However, in the future it may well be that there is a cost argument for the more precise selection of patients for individual treatments.

Bladder outflow obstruction
Techniques for measuring obstruction

A simple flow rate with an adequate voided volume will identify with some confidence a large proportion of men with obstruction (Roerhborn *et al.* 1995). Eighty-eight per cent of patients with flow rates <10 ml/sec and 68 per cent of those with <15 ml/sec are shown to be obstructed by formal urodynamic testing. Provided the measurements are taken with care using two or more measures and adequate voided volume, the use of simple flow rates is indicated for the majority of patients in whom all other factors point to the presence of obstruction and the treatment is going to be non-invasive.

The measurement of the detrusor pressure together with the urinary flow rate has been used for many years in the investigation of lower urinary tract function. Advanced urodynamic tests are specifically indicated for the investigation of complex urological problems in neurological and paediatric patients. Such studies were regarded in the past as being too invasive for routine use in common conditions. Recently, a better understanding of the pathophysiology of obstruction as well as improvements in study techniques and equipment have made it possible to consider the more frequent use of these investigations in men with LUTS. The techniques for

Table 3.4 The relationship of prostate volume (PV) and peak flow rate to the incidence of urodynamically defined outflow obstruction

110 men		Flow rate (ml/sec)		
		All	>10	<10
PV (ml)	All	68	66	88
	<30	60	48	79
	30–45	67	67	94
	>45	82	78	90

performing the test have become more standardised and guidelines from the International Continence Society are very helpful in establishing a unit which is able to produce consistently good quality studies (Griffiths *et al.* 1997; Abrams *et al.* 1998). The study is now usually performed with a double lumen tube of 8F or less passed through the urethra into the bladder. One lumen is used for filling and the pressure can be recorded through the other by connection to a simple transducer allowing repeated measurements of the pressure–flow relationship. At the same time pressure is recorded from a balloon placed in the rectum. When the rectal pressure is subtracted from the bladder pressure, a measure of the pressure developed by the detrusor muscle is obtained. The urethral catheter is narrow enough that voiding can occur around it – although the flow will be less than in a free flow rate, it is still representative of normal voiding (Walker *et al.* 1998). It is important that the test is performed in an as friendly and relaxed environment as possible in order to avoid inhibition of flow and a consequent overestimation of obstruction. For pressure–flow studies in men with LUTS it is not necessary to have complicated X-ray screening and voiding can be in private. The important measurement from the study is the detrusor pressure at maximum flow, by which the diagnosis of obstruction is made in most classifications. In addition, it is sometimes relevant to measure either the minimal voiding pressure or the pressure at the beginning of flow. A simple graphical trace of pressure versus flow is a useful aid to the interpretation of the study. Care should be taken to avoid relying on the automatic figures presented by modern urodynamic machines as there are many potential sources of error. Simple manual calculation is all that is needed for most interpretations (Manieri *et al.* 1998). Currently, there is considerable research activity in trying to find ways of measuring the degree of obstruction by non-invasive methods; although this remains in development, it is likely that in the future new ways of looking at this problem will be identified.

It has taken a considerable time to find ways of making sense of the complex information contained within the voiding phase of the study. Standardisation of terms and definitions of obstruction have finally been agreed. By and large, the various classifications of obstruction have now reached a consensus. Most of the well-known nomograms (Schäfer, Abrams-Griffiths, ICS) are in agreement as to the definition of the obstructed patient (Abrams *et al.* 1995). There remains a grey area where the patient is classified as 'equivocal', and the significance for a patient who falls into this region is very uncertain; repeated testing may be necessary to establish whether or not the finding is significant (Javle *et al.* 1996; Abrams *et al.* 1998).

The significance of urodynamically defined obstruction

Much of the controversy regarding the use of urodynamic studies in the management of the man with LUTS stems from the long and complex discussions which were held some years ago as to the best method of defining obstruction. In part, this arises from the fact that many healthy older men are known from population-based studies to have low flow rates. In a volunteer study of asymptomatic older men we found that 20 per cent were obstructed by the Abrams-Griffiths nomogram (Walker *et al.* 1997b). Consequently, it is difficult to know how to define 'normal' levels. Should 'normal' be regarded as a man without prostatic enlargement, or of a certain age, or after a disobliterating procedure such as a TURP, or even the voiding pressures in a woman? It is thus essential that interpretation of the pressure–flow study takes into account both the symptoms that the patient experiences and the anatomical evidence of obstruction.

We can identify a group of men in whom we have no doubt that abnormally high voiding pressures only result in a low flow and in whom we can predict with confidence that a reduction in the outflow resistance will produce an improvement at least in the urodynamic state. However, any man over the age of 20 years would notice a change in voiding on removal of the prostatic inner zones and division of the bladder neck, with an improvement in flow rate, which is usually regarded as being beneficial. It is thus difficult to interpret the significance of equivocal obstruction in the context of symptom change in patients after treatment. Of more importance is the issue of whether treatment of a truly unobstructed man by prostatectomy will produce any benefit. It is generally agreed that the outcome is worse when patients are selected on the basis of symptoms alone, although evidence to support this is now hard to find but recent work has shown that some unobstructed symptomatic patients will have benefit from a TURP. What can be stated in confidence is that men should not undergo treatment for obstruction alone, as natural history studies strongly suggest that many will have the same symptoms many years later, and few will come to any harm in terms of developing complications, if left without treatment (Garraway *et al.* 1991).

Measuring the degree of obstruction is also of importance in deciding which treatment to advise: some therapies are unlikely to reduce obstruction very greatly and indeed some treatments may in the short term make the situation worse. If a man is shown on pressure–flow studies to have a very obstructed bladder, then some form of treatment which produces a substantial increase in diameter of the prostatic lumen is needed in order to restore normal voiding mechanics. Such treatments at present include conventional TURP and open prostatectomy as well as new laser methods of adenoma enucleation. Lesser degrees of obstruction, on the other hand, may be treated by techniques which do not produce a large cavity and may also spare the bladder neck and the consequences of retrograde ejaculation. Such treatments include those which rely on heating of the prostate without immediate tissue destruction and less satisfactory methods of gland destruction such as laser vaporisation.

Other information available from the pressure–flow study

Further information regarding the type of obstruction may be available from the pressure–flow study. It has been postulated that there is more than one pattern of obstruction (Schäfer 1985). The best explanation of this is by the CHESS classification, which disassociates the slope of the linear PURR from the footpoint (Hofner *et al.* 1995). Patients may have either a steep slope or a high footpoint pressure or indeed a combination of both. These two patterns of compressive and constrictive obstruction may be important in determining outcome after treatment (Figure 3.4). The prime example of this is the use of the low-energy transurethral microwave therapy system from Edap Technomed, which uses an applicator with a hot point 10 mm below the bladder neck. It is therefore possible to create a large cavity in the prostatic urethra but not to change the bladder neck configuration (Tubaro *et al.* 1995; Hofner *et al.* 1998). Evidence from retrospective studies shows that patients with constrictive pattern have a considerably better outcome than those with a predominantly compressive pattern. The same consideration does not apply to TURP where, while the bulk of the prostate is removed, the bladder neck is opened simultaneously either by resection or, in some surgeons' hands, by a deliberate incision. A hypothesis can be made that the element of obstruction that accounts for the high footpoint of the linear PURR can be ascribed to bladder neck performance, whereas the slope of the PURR is more a reflection of the obstruction within the prostate (Schäfer 1985).

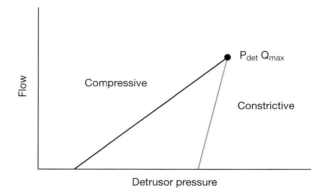

Figure 3.4 Demonstration of two different patterns of urodynamic obstruction by linear PURR with the same $P_{det} Q_{max}$. In constrictive obstruction the pressure remains high throughout the voiding cycle, whereas in compressive obstruction there are times when voiding pressures are low

While such a hypothesis remains to be proven, there are obviously some patients in whom a treatment which affects the bladder neck alone fails to relieve the obstruction completely, and others where effective treatment of the prostate adenoma is insufficient. Such considerations are of importance if the full benefits of minimally invasive therapy are to be made use of and the treatment-related damage to sexual function is to be minimised.

Bladder function in the man with LUTS

In the man with LUTS there are three distinct changes which can occur in bladder function:

- the bladder contraction becomes less powerful and as a result develops low pressure voiding with a low flow;
- the bladder develops abnormal function in the storage phase, such as unstable contractions or sensory urgency (Hald *et al.* 1995);
- hypertrophy of the detrusor occurs in compensation for the obstruction.

Each abnormality may well influence the decision regarding treatment. In practice, it is usually the weak bladder that causes most difficulty in terms of diagnosis; yet the overactive bladder is the most difficult problem to treat. Bladder wall hypertrophy is the measurement to make. Each abnormality will be considered, although it is the strength of the detrusor that defines the domain of the classification in which the patient lies.

Detrusor power

One of the problems for the measurement of bladder function is to establish the strength of the detrusor muscle. On a simple level, we often assume that the post-void residual volume (PVR) is an indicator of the ability of the bladder to contract efficiently (Abrams & Griffiths 1979). Measurement of PVR is simple and commonly performed as a baseline investigation in men with symptoms, although the significance of the information in terms of outflow function is poorly understood. PVR is seldom used as a primary outcome measure in therapeutic clinical trials, although we certainly expect a reduction in an effective treatment. One of the main problems with PVR is that the values obtained from a single measurement may not be representative. A number of values from voids of different volumes are needed to get some feel for the true situation as might be experienced by the patient in normal life. Unfortunately, there is no easy method of measuring detrusor contraction even using complex urodynamic studies. Several methods have been proposed: the p iso measured during forced stopping of the flow, the projected isometric pressure derived from $P_{det} Q_{max}$ and more sophisticated power measures derived from the whole pressure–flow sequence using a calculated reduction in volume for a given amount of bladder work (Abrams *et al.* 1995). The simplest method is to use the classes of detrusor contraction on the Schäfer nomogram. The validity of these measures is uncertain and their use limited to research practice.

The clinical significance of 'weak' detrusor

The problem in interpretation of the findings of either a large residual urine volume or complex urodynamic measures is that there are many different causes of any apparent weakness, at least some of which are independent of the presence of outflow obstruction. It is well recognised that impaired detrusor function can occur as a result of ageing without any evidence of outflow obstruction. To many clinicians, the presence of significant residual urine represents a decompensated bladder where the amount of work available runs out before the bladder has emptied. However, the relationship between bladder contractility and residual urine remains uncertain. It is assumed by many that the residual volume is a result of reduced detrusor contractility, although there is no evidence to support this. Therefore an increased residual volume does not necessarily imply a failing bladder and many patients continue to void without significant problems but with very large residual volumes (Bruskewitz *et al.* 1982; Srinaulnad 1999). How the detrusor function continues to change in the face of obstruction is unknown. In some, the bladder remains compensated but in others there is a loss of function with a decrease in power and it is presumed that it is these patients who will be at risk of an acute retention. In consequence, it is often difficult to advise the patient with LUTS and significant residual urine as to the future risks of acute retention, often a concern of considerable importance to the patient. In practice, where there is demonstrable obstruction and a large residual volume, some form of definitive treatment is usually advised. Additional support for this decision is given by information suggesting a weak detrusor from the pressure–flow study. It is certainly true that the complications of BOO arise from either an increased residual volume (infection, stone formations, etc.) or a failing detrusor (acute retention).

Measurement of bladder function during filling

Most men with LUTS are more concerned with the storage symptoms of frequency and urgency than they are with voiding symptoms of hesitancy, flow and emptying (Akino *et al.* 1996; Blaivas 1996). Unfortunately, the symptoms associated with storage are not particularly well understood and notoriously difficult to treat. The filling phase of the urodynamic study may be regarded as the least physiological part of the test. Bladder-filling is generally performed at rates far greater than it occurs naturally, and the tests used to provoke an unstable bladder contraction, such as changing from standing to lying or altering rates of filling, are poorly understood and not easily reproducible. Generally, a standard filling rate of 50 ml/min is used. It is important that every unit devises its own strategy for the filling phase and does not change the technique between studies. It is of crucial importance that the investigators reporting the study understand that the occurrence of a rise in detrusor pressure during filling, in the absence of any sensation, is not defined as an unstable contraction and for the time being should be regarded as artefactual. For the present, a rise in pressure of 15 cm/H_2O during an abnormal detrusor contraction is regarded as significant. Repeated filling studies may be needed to evaluate the suspicion of an overactive bladder. Ambulatory studies may be of use in arguable cases but these are difficult to perform and require more complex and expensive equipment. Still more obscure in the interpretation of the filling phase is the assessment of sensory phenomena in the absence of changes in detrusor pressure. There is no doubt that sensory urgency (i.e. the desire to pass urine in the absence of an unstable contraction at low filling volume) is poorly understood and difficult to measure, yet common, and often appears to be related to the symptoms experienced by the patient. More information as to the sensory component of the voiding reflex is urgently required to make sense of our patients' symptoms. In the mean time a simple subjective assessment of the presence of sensory urgency is a useful part of the report of the UDS which only the person performing the test can comment on. The importance in training the staff performing the urodynamic studies and quality control is most evident in the evaluation of the filling characteristics.

The clinical significance of the overactive detrusor

Clinical experience indicates that many men who have unstable bladders on urodynamic studies do not fare well after treatment. The finding of an overactive bladder in an older man should always prompt the clinician to consider other diseases that could be the cause. In particular, the risk of malignancy should be excluded by adequate cytological examination of the bladder and, if appropriate, cystoscopy and bladder biopsy. A more likely diagnosis is the presence of some form of occult neurological disease, which may be present in addition to the obstruction. is although with time their voiding symptoms often do settle. It is open to question what proportion of bladder instability seen in association with BOO is due entirely to compensatory changes in the detrusor. In practice, at least a third of patients with LUTS undergoing comprehensive urodynamic testing will have some evidence of bladder overactivity. More men will have evidence of sensory abnormalities, particularly in the younger age group. In terms of treatment the finding of increased bladder sensation should serve as a warning that relief of obstruction may not produce a complete resolution of urinary frequency.

Hypertrophy of the bladder

An increase in bladder mass is not in itself a cause of symptoms but the measurement of hypertrophy may be of interest in the diagnosis of significant outflow obstruction. Hypertrophy can also occur in other conditions, such as neuropathic bladder, and it is also said to occur in women in the presence of bladder instability. Recent studies of bladder-wall thickness measurements by ultrasound imaging have shown good diagnostic specificity for obstruction in men with LUTS (Manieri *et al.* 1998; Ochiai & Kojima 1998). The ultrasound study should be performed on a bladder of known volume and without previous catheterisation, which may thicken the bladder wall by mucosal changes. Three measurements of the thickness of the bladder wall are taken using a simple suprapubic scan and averaged. A simple mathematical formula can be applied to calculate the weight of bladder muscle (Ochiai & Kojima 1998). The clinical significance of bladder wall thickness or bladder mass measurements is shown in Table 3.5.

Table 3.5 The relationship of prostate volume (PV) and bladder neck steepness (BNS) to the incidence of urodynamically defined outflow obstruction and mean values of URA and Schäfer class. Small prostates with a steep bladder neck (≥40 mm) have a 100 per cent incidence of obstruction

PV (ml)	BNS (mm)	No. men	Obstr. (%)	URA	Schäfer class
<40	<15	41	58.5	38.5	2.8
<40	≥15	10	100	47.7	3.9
≥40	<15	14	92.9	44.1	3.6
≥40	≥15	26	92.3	52.4	4.1

Benign prostatic enlargement
Techniques for measuring prostatic size

The simplest investigation measurement of prostatic size is by digital rectal examination (DRE); however, digital examination only measures two of three dimensions and in larger prostates it often underestimates size. Furthermore, there is no agreed system for recording the results of the measurement; is the stated value the total gland volume or the expected resection weight? Many clinicians simply state whether the prostate is small, enlarged or very large. Even such simple statements are difficult to define. Additional confirmation of prostate size is useful. For many years, assessment of the lower urinary tract included upper tract imaging by the intravenous urogram. Previous generations of urologists were skilled at interpreting the pre- and post-voiding bladder views to help them decide on the size of the prostate and the suitability of a patient for prostatectomy. The advent of access to sophisticated ultrasound devices in the clinical setting by others than radiologists gives the possibility to image the lower urinary tract in detail, routinely. The urologist now has an opportunity to investigate the relationship between structure and function. Prostate volume can be measured from images of the bladder obtained by suprapubic scanning and the accuracy is said to be reasonable (Prassopoulos *et al.* 1996). However, few radiological reports include this information and in some men it is difficult to see the margins of the prostate or to measure the length of the gland.

The most important tool for measurement of prostatic size is the transrectal ultrasound probe, which can be used to obtain detailed measurements of size and information about the shape and the internal architecture of the prostate. Other methods of measuring prostatic size include MRI and CT scan. Complex cross-sectional imaging has the advantage that three-dimensional reconstruction can be performed more easily than by ultrasound, which requires the use of fixed external reference points for the transducer. However, issues of radiation protection and cost prevent these investigations being used for prostatic volume measurement except in the most complex research projects. Further discussion will be restricted to the information from transrectal ultrasound scanning.

Technical considerations of transrectal ultrasound screening

Unfortunately, the development of transrectal sonography has been dominated by its application in the diagnosis and assessment of prostate cancer. The probes were designed with biopsy in mind rather than the determination of the spatial relationships of the prostate to the urethra and bladder. The ideal rectal probe for the study of patients with LUTS has yet to be produced but a linear array in the sagittal plane probably gives the best definition of the prostatic urethra and bladder neck structures. Transverse imaging can be obtained by sector probes that ideally should have a wide-enough sweep to encompass the whole width of a large gland. It is important that the planes of view are obtained in strict orthogonal relationship so that the prostate volume can be measured by a three-dimensional technique according to strict geometrical rules. The choice of the frequency for the transducer is important for imaging in patients with BPH. A lower frequency of between 4 and 6 MHz is necessary to define the anterior border of a very large prostate, whereas higher-frequency probes may be more suitable for detailed imaging of the peripheral zone in the investigation of cancer.

The technique of rectal ultrasound scanning is relatively easy to master, although proper training is essential for clinicians unfamiliar with ultrasonography in general. The bladder should contain a small amount of urine to define the superior border of the prostate. Often the scan is performed after micturition so that the residual volume can be calculated at the same time. If linear array probes are used, the discomfort from a diagnostic ultrasound is minimal. More discomfort is experienced if an end fire multi-plane probe is used because angulation on the anus is required to obtain transverse images of the prostate. With practice, a diagnostic prostatic ultrasound need not take much longer than a careful DRE. Attention to detail and a standard technique should be employed with a clear system of nomenclature to describe the different areas and lobes of the prostate. Difficulties are often encountered in obtaining accurate measurement in the post-operative patient where there is a large cavity in the centre of the gland. A few patients have disease of the anus and rectum, which makes diagnostic ultrasound uncomfortable. The test is otherwise well tolerated and has no significant adverse effects.

Measurements from transrectal prostatic ultrasound imaging

Prostate volume is the most important measurement in the man with LUTS. Measurement of the total volume is usually sufficient but there may be additional information to be gained by the measurement of the transition zone volume (Kurita *et al.* 1996). A number of different techniques of measurement have been proposed. The most accurate is with planimetry and the integration of the area of the prostate on images taken at set intervals. Planimetry is clumsy and difficult to perform quickly. Most people use a simple three-dimensional calculation multiplying the length by the width by the A-P diameter and dividing the product by a factor (usually 2). Several authors have calculated the transition zone index (the ratio between total volume and transition zone volume) and claimed it to be a more accurate predictor of both symptom status and obstruction (Kurita *et al.* 1996; Witjes *et al.* 1997). There is probably little to be gained by this more complex technique.

Another interesting measurement is that of the presumed circular area where the shape of the prostate is compared to the volume and seems to have a useful relationship with the obstruction status of the patient (Kojima *et al.* 1997).

The relationship between prostatic volume and other parameters in the BPH patient

The significance of a large prostate is shown in Table 3.6. In this series of 151 men with LUTS, just two-thirds were obstructed by urodynamic criteria. In the 38 with total prostate volume of 45 ml or more, 84 per cent were obstructed. Perhaps more importantly, there is no similar relationship between those with small (<26 ml) and medium (27–45 ml) volumes in terms of symptoms and only minor differences in flow rate. Interestingly, the residual volume seems to increase with size of the prostate. In practice, these data can be used to predict the presence of obstruction using measures of volume and flow rate as shown in Table 3.5. Men with prostates of less than 30 ml and flow rates of greater than 10 ml/sec have only a 50 per cent likelihood of being obstructed, as opposed to those with prostates larger than 45 and flow rates less than 10 ml/sec, of whom 90 per cent are obstructed. At the least, this information may be used to select a group of patients who should have further physiological testing by urodynamic studies to confirm obstruction before they are subjected to any surgical procedure.

Table 3.6 The relationship of prostate volume (PV) to other measurements of lower urinary tract function

	No.	MSS	Vol. ml	PFR ml/sec	PVR ml	P_{det} Q_{max}	Obstr (%)
All	151	12.1	38	10.8	96	77	68
PV (ml)							
<26	45	12.1	20	11.2	86	68	62
26–45	68	11.6	35	11.0	94	76	63
>45	38	12.7	64	9.9	112	89	84

The importance of prostatic volume in treatment selection

Knowledge of the prostate volume is possibly the most important factor for the planning of treatment. Most commonly, the information is used in selecting the appropriate surgical procedure. Patients in whom obstruction has been identified with small prostates may be suitable for simple bladder neck incision or transurethral incision of prostate. The volume of larger prostates may be used in planning transurethral resection (Aus *et al.* 1994). For instance, knowing that a prostate is in the range of 60–80 g in size will ensure that enough time is allowed for a big resection and perhaps will signal that it is not a suitable operation for a junior surgeon with little experience of TURP. If the prostate is known to be of an even larger size, the patient can be warned that an open procedure may well be indicated and this may change the way in which he views the need for treatment. There are obvious advantages in knowing that an open procedure will be needed in terms of preparing both the patient and the operating theatre. Similarly, transurethral vaporisation of the prostate is generally considered to be best reserved only for prostates of moderate size because the rate of tissue removal is relatively slow.

Prostate volume has been proven to be of importance in the selection of the patient for medical therapy. It has been shown that finasteride therapy is only really effective in patients with larger prostates presumably because an absolute decrease in prostate size is necessary to produce any relief of obstruction (Boyle *et al.* 1996). The planning of tissue-destructive techniques using heating is essential and knowledge of both the size and position of the adenoma may exclude certain treatments. For instance, transurethral microwave thermotherapy must not be undertaken in patients with very small glands for fear that the irradiative heat field may damage the external sphincter or rectum. Furthermore, small prostates do not heat up as well, probably because the blood supply is greater than usual. Certain patterns and size of adenomatous growth may be more suitable for the various laser techniques.

Other useful information from transrectal prostatic ultrasound

A new concept for the analysis of prostatic images is that of bladder neck steepness or the angulation of the urethra at the junction of the peripheral and central zones of the prostate. For the experienced ultrasonographer it is easy to identify the junction, which is also the position of the veru montanum. Measurements are made between this point and the rectal wall and between the internal meatus and the rectal wall. Subtracting the two values gives an indication of the steepness of the bladder neck (see Figure 3.5). The information obtained is similar to that seen by placing a cystoscope at the veru montanum and looking towards the bladder. In small prostates it is easy to identify the various landmarks but in large adenomas the internal meatus may be difficult to see. Care must be taken not to distort the anterior wall of the rectum by placing pressure on it with the probe.

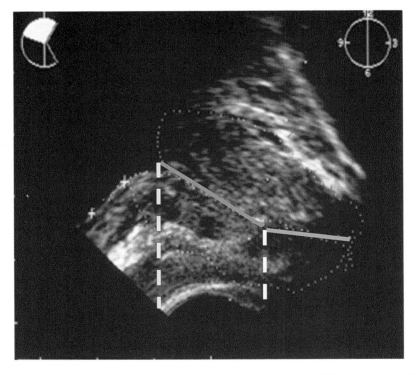

Figure 3.5 The curvature of the bladder neck can be described by measuring the distance from the bladder neck to rectal wall (BNR) and subtracting from this the veru montanum to rectal distance (VR)

Bladder neck steepness has been shown to be related to the incidence of obstruction particularly in small prostates (see Table 3.5, on p.55) (Trucchi *et al.* 1998). In the future it may be possible by careful analysis of the prostatic ultrasound to identify groups of patients where obstruction is likely and there is no need for pressure–flow studies before recommending surgical intervention. Recent work by our unit also suggests that the internal sphincter muscle can be identified and perhaps abnormalities such as hypertrophy can be diagnosed, although this remains a matter for research.

Other important information from images of the bladder neck may be available, including the identification of the middle lobe. The identification of an isolated middle lobe of the prostate will certainly encourage the urologist to believe that a TURP will improve voiding (el Din *et al.* 1996). The middle lobe may be identified by the suprapubic and transrectal ultrasound scan. The lobar anatomy may be difficult to identify if the bladder is completely empty or if the gland is very large. In the patient who has undergone a failed obliterative procedure, the residual 'lumps' of prostatic tissue prolapsing into the prostatic urethra may help confirm the impression from other investigations that a redo TURP will be of benefit. In the evaluation of post-prostatectomy stress pattern incontinence, a definite defect in the sphincter may be seen and generally the limits of the resection can be seen to have been too distal anteriorly.

Qualitative information from images of the prostate is less specific than the information from the measurements of volume and bladder neck steepness; however, it often has practical use in deciding the best treatment for individuals with confusing symptoms or results from urodynamic studies. There is debate as to the significance of echo-reflective material within the prostate (Doble & Carter 1989). At least some of the echogenic structures must be regarded as normal. In simple BPH there are often corpora amylacea within the ducts at the margin of the central and peripheral prostate. These are well recognised during TURP as released once the resection has reached the posterior surgical capsule. Other echodensities are seen on the prostatic urethra and seem to be associated with irritable voiding. There can be little doubt that massive calcification seen within the prostate (usually after previous surgery) is abnormal and may contribute to the symptoms (Sant *et al.* 1984). In a recent review of our patients undergoing comprehensive investigation, we found a significant association between the presence of echodensities and bladder instability. The presence of echodense areas within the prostate gave a nearly threefold increased risk of instability or sensory bladder phenomena. However, no discrete pattern of echodensity or distribution within the prostate was particularly associated with abnormal bladder function. It would seem logical that these changes are indicative of a sensory phenomenon arising within the prostate affecting the storage mechanism of the bladder. Further work is needed to clarify whether there is any therapeutic relevance to this observation.

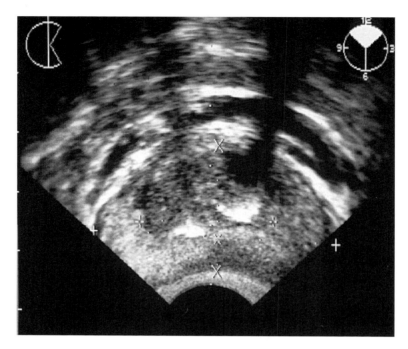

Figure 3.6 Gross calcification of the prostate in man with multiple symptoms suggestive of both obstruction and prostatitis

Lower urinary tract symptoms (LUTS)

Techniques for further investigation

Further investigations to explain the cause of LUTS are often performed in the initial stages as a process of exclusion of other diagnoses. The measurement of symptoms with the use of symptoms scores is now firmly established. Self-assessment by the patient with the International Prostate Symptoms Score (IPSS) is widely accepted as the best tool. Other symptoms scores are available; some more detailed, some filled in by the health care worker rather than the patient (Barry *et al.* 1992). Of most importance is the assessment of 'bother'. This single question in the IPSS is the most relevant to modern clinical practice as we accept that treatment is indicated only if the patient is disturbed by his symptoms (Jacobsen *et al.* 1993). More detailed assessments of quality of life are available but are only used for research purposes.

A number of other specific investigations may be of use in clarifying whether LUTS in an individual are due to BPE and BOO and consequently amenable to treatment by relief of prostatic obstruction. These include the use of a detailed frequency–volume chart, cystoscopy and a detailed microbiological survey. While many aspects of these investigations remain outside the scope of this chapter, some will be discussed briefly in the light of establishing the diagnosis and cause of LUTS. The investigations are of particular importance in establishing whether filling phase symptoms and sensory abnormalities found on the urodynamic studies are as a result of obstruction or not. In general it is in the younger patients that these further investigations of symptoms may be necessary.

Frequency–volume chart

Many patients presenting with LUTS are elderly and have other conditions that may cause abnormalities of urine production. These may be identified by having the patient keep an accurate record of the volume of urine passed and the time. Identification of nocturnal polyuria and drug-related diuresis may reveal the true cause of symptoms (Chapple 1993). Some would argue that all patients should fill in such a chart for consideration at the first clinic appointment but, as abnormalities of urine production are relatively rare, I recommend using this only when there are doubts as to the real cause of the symptoms.

Cystoscopy

In the past it was customary to perform a cystoscopy in most, if not all, patients before deciding on a surgical intervention. While there are certain visual clues as to the presence of obstruction, these can now be obtained by non-invasive imaging. The role for cystoscopy in current clinical practice is the exclusion of other causes of obstruction and symptoms (Roehrborn *et al.* 1995). In general most cystoscopy is undertaken as a local anaesthetic procedure with a flexible instrument. Flexible cystoscopy is sufficient to identify urethral strictures and gross pathology of the bladder. Local anaesthetic cystoscopy has the disadvantage of not being able to measure the maximum bladder capacity and it is perhaps more difficult to identify the prostatic urethral anatomy without high flow of irrigant. Biopsies can be taken but are sometimes inadequate for histological diagnosis.

It is debatable in which patients a cystoscopy is indicated. I recommend a flexible cystoscopy in patients with a flat flow curve that might suggest a stricture. Where there are inflammatory cells in the urine together with marked sensory symptoms or small voided volumes, I recommend general anaesthetic cystoscopy to obtain an adequate biopsy material of the bladder and to measure the maximum bladder capacity. I also take the opportunity of performing a vigorous prostatic massage, which can occasionally help patients with inflammatory prostatic disease.

Microbiological survey

The many and varied conditions of prostatitis frequently cause a diagnostic dilemma in the investigation of the man with LUTS. Few precise diagnostic tools are available (NIH 1995). The presence of white cells in the absence of overt infection in the mid-stream urine specimen may alert one to the possibility that there is inflammatory disease within the prostate. Currently the definitive test for prostatitis is the Stamey–Meares test examining the expressed prostatic secretions and post-massage urine for both white cells and infection. Determining whether there is prostatic infection is particularly important when the patient is being investigated for recurrent urinary tract infection in association with symptoms, possibly resulting from BOO. If there is chronic bacterial prostatitis, appropriate and sustained antibacterial therapy is likely to have a much better outcome than surgical intervention. Patients with significant levels of pain in association with LUTS are also more likely to have chronic prostatitis and again surgical intervention has a dismal success rate in relieving them of the symptoms that trouble them most. However, some authorities have argued that, in the presence of gross calcification of the prostate, surgical removal may help some patients with chronic relapsing prostatitis.

Conclusions

Whatever strategy for the investigation of the BPH patient a particular unit decides upon, a comprehensive plan of treatment for each type of patient described by the extended classification shown in Figure 3.2 is needed. In general the patient who does not fit into the central zone of the diagram (Figure 3.1) will need at least some additional investigations to try to decide whether treatment is needed and if so which of the many modalities available is likely to be of benefit. As an example: the man with LUTS, a large prostate but minimal obstruction and a healthy bladder would seem to be an ideal candidate for finasteride therapy in the first instance. Whereas a man with obstruction, a normal bladder and few if any symptoms would be placed on a watchful-waiting programme. Many questions remain about the relationship between symptoms, obstruction, prostatic enlargement and bladder function. However, the judicious use of more complicated investigation for patients in whom the symptoms and findings do not obviously fit into the familiar pattern is both rewarding and often fascinating.

References

Aarnink RG, Beerlage HP, de la Rosette JJ, Debruyne FM & Wijkstra H (1998). Transrectal ultrasound of the prostate: innovations and future applications. [Review] [76 refs]. *Journal of Urology* **159**, 1568–79.

Abrams P (1995). Objective evaluation of outlet obstruction. *Br J Urol* 1995; **76**, 11–5.

Abrams P & Griffiths D (1979). The assessment of prostatic obstruction from urodynamic measurements and from residual urine. *Br J Urol* **51**, 129–134.

Abrams P, Bruskewitz RC, de-la-Rosette J *et al.* (1995). The diagnosis of bladder outlet obstruction: urodynamics. In *The 3rd International Consultation on Benign Prostatic Hyperplasia (BPH)* (ed. ATK Cockett, S Khoury, Y Aso *et al.*), pp. 297–368. SCI, Jersey, Channel Islands.

Abrams P, Buzelin JM, Griffiths D *et al.* (1998). The urodynamic assessment of lower urinary tract symptoms. In *Proceedings of the 4th International Consultation on Benign Prostatic Hyperplasia (BPH)* (ed. L Denis, D Griffiths, S Khoury *et al.*), pp.323–77. Health Publication Ltd, Jersey (UK).

Akino H, Gobara M & Okada K (1996). Bladder dysfunction in patients with benign prostatic hyperplasia: relevance of cystometry as prognostic indicator of the outcome after prostatectomy. *Int J Urol* **3**, 441–7.

Aus G, Bergdahl S, Hugosson J & Norlen L (1994). Volume determinations of the whole prostate and of adenomas by transrectal ultrasound in patients with clinically benign prostatic hyperplasia: correlation of resected weight, blood loss and duration of operation. *Br J Urol* **73**, 659–63.

Barry MJ, Fowler FJJ, O'Leary MP, Bruskewitz RC, Holtgrewe HL & Mebust WK (1992). Correlation of the American Urological Association symptom index with self-administered versions of the Madsen-Iversen, Boyarsky and Maine Medical Assessment Program symptom indexes. Measurement Committee of the American Urological Association. *Journal of Urology* **148**, 1558–63.

Blaivas JG (1996). Obstructive uropathy in the male. *Urol Clin North Am* **23**, 373–84.

Boyle P, Gould AL & Roehrborn CG (1996). Prostate volume predicts the outcome of treatment of benign prostatic hyperplasia with finasteride: meta-analysis of randomized clinical trials. *Urology* **48**, 398–405.

Bruskewitz RC, Iversen P & Madsen PO (1982). Value of postvoid residual urine determination in evaluation of prostatism. *Urology* **20**, 602–4.

Chapple CR (1993). Correlation of symptomatology, urodynamics, morphology and size of the prostate in benign prostatic hyperplasia. *Curr Opinion in Urology* **3**, 5–9.

Comiter CV, Sullivan MP, Schacterle RS, Cohen LH & Valla SV (1997). Urodynamic risk factors for renal dysfunction in men with obstructive and nonobstructive voiding dysfunction. *J Urol* **158**, 181–5.

de-Wildt MJ, Debruyne FM & de-la-Rosette JJ (1996). High-energy transurethral microwave thermotherapy: a thermoablative treatment for benign prostatic obstruction. *Urology* **48**, 416–23.

Doble A & Carter SStC (1989). Ultrasonographic findings in prostatitis. *Urol Clin North Am* **16**, 751–763.

el Din KE, de Wildt MJ, Rosier PF, Wijkstra H, Debruyne FM & de la Rosette JJ (1996). The correlation between urodynamic and cystoscopic findings in elderly men with voiding complaints. *Journal of Urology* **155**, 1018–22.

Garraway WM, Collins GN & Lee RJ (1991). High prevalence of benign prostatic hypertrophy in the community. *Lancet* **338**, 469–71.

Griffiths D, Höfner K, van Maastrigt R, Rollema HJ & Gleason DM (1997). Standardisation of terminology of lower urinary tract function: pressure-flow studies of voiding, urethral resistance, and urethral obstruction. *Neurourol Urodyn* **16**, 1–18.

Hald T (1989). Urodynamics in benign prostatic hyperplasia: a survey. *Prostate – Supplement* **2**, 69–77.

Hald T, Brading A, Elbadawi A *et al.* (1995). The urinary bladder in obstruction and ageing. In *The 3rd International Consultation on Benign Prostatic Hyperplasia (BPH)* (ed. ATK Cockett, S Khoury, Y Aso *et al.*), pp.167–254. SCI, Jersey, Channel Islands.

Hofner K, Kramer AE, Tan HK, Krah H & Jonas U (1995). CHESS classification of bladder-outflow obstruction. A consequence in the discussion of current concepts. *World J Urol* **13**, 59–64.

Hofner K, Tubaro A, de la Rosette JJ & Carter SS (1998). Analysis of outcome after thermotherapy using different classifications of bladder outlet obstruction. *Neurourol Urodyn* **17**, 109–20.

Jacobsen SJ, Girman CJ, Guess HA, Panser LA, Chute CG, Oesterling JE & Lieber MM (1993). Natural history of prostatism: factors associated with discordance between frequency and bother of urinary symptoms. *Urology* **42**, 663–71.

Javle P, Jenkins SA, West C & Parsons KF (1996). Quantification of voiding dysfunction in patients awaiting transurethral prostatectomy. *J Urol* **156**, 1014–18.

Jensen KM, Jorgensen JB & Mogensen P (1988). Urodynamics in prostatism. I. Prognostic value of uroflowmetry. *Scandinavian Journal of Urology & Nephrology* **22**, 109–17.

Jepsen JV & Bruskewitz RC (1998). Comprehensive patient evaluation for benign prostatic hyperplasia. [Review] [37 refs]. *Urology* **51**(4A Suppl.), 13–8.

Kojima M, Ochiai A, Naya Y, Ukimura O, Watanabe M & Watanabe H (1997). Correlation of presumed circle area ratio with infravesical obstruction in men with lower urinary tract symptoms. *Urology* **50**, 548–55.

Kurita Y, Ushiyama T, Suzuki K, Fujita K & Kawabe K (1996). Transition zone ratio and prostate-specific antigen density: the index of response of benign prostatic hypertrophy to an alpha blocker. *Int J Urol* **3**, 361–6.

McConnell JD, Barry MJ & Bruskewitz RC (1994). Benign prostatic hyperplasia: diagnosis and treatment. Agency for Health Care Policy and Research. *Clin Pract Guide/Quick Ref Guide Clin* (8), 1–17.

Manieri C, Carter SStC, Romano G, Trucchi A, Valenti M & Tubaro A (1998). The diagnosis of bladder outlet obstruction in men by ultrasound measurement of bladder wall thickness. *J Urol* **159**, 761–5.

Neal DE, Ramsden PD & Sharples L (1989). Outcome of prostatectomy. *BMJ* **299**, 762–7.

[NIH] National Institutes of Health (1995). *Summary statement.* Presented at National Institutes of Health/National Institute of Diabetes and Digestive and Kidney Disease. Disease Workshop on Chronic Prostatitis.

Ochiai A & Kojima M (1998). Correlation of ultrasound-estimated bladder weight with ultrasound appearance of the prostate and postvoid residual urine in men with lower urinary tract symptoms. *Urology* **51**, 722–9.

Prassopoulos P, Charoulakis N, Anezinis P, Daskalopoulos G, Cranidis A & Gourtsoyiannis N (1996). Suprapubic versus transrectal ultrasonography in assessing the volume of the prostate and the transition zone in patients with benign prostatic hyperplasia. *Abdominal Imaging* **21**, 75–7.

Roehrborn CG, Andersen JT, Correa R *et al.* (1995). Initial diagnostic evaluation of men with lower urinary tract symptoms. In *The 3rd International Consultation on Benign Prostatic Hyperplasia (BPH)* (ed. ATK Cockett, S Khoury, Y Aso *et al.*), pp.167–254. SCI, Jersey, Channel Islands.

Sant GR, Heaney JA & Meares EM (1984). 'Radical' transurethral prostatic resection in the management of chronic abacterial prostatitis. *J Urol* **131**, 184A.

Schäfer W (1985). Urethral resistance? Urodynamic concepts of physiological and pathological bladder outlet function during voiding. *Neurourol Urodyn* **4**, 161.

Srinaulnad S, Carter SS, Renzetti R & Tubaro A (1999). Post void residual and bladder power factors in men with LUTS. *Br J Urol* **31**(Suppl).

Steers WD & Zorn B (1995). Benign prostatic hyperplasia. [Review] [181 refs]. *Disease-A-Month* **41**, 437–97.

Thomas AW & Abrams P (1998). Patient selection: the value of pressure-flow urodynamics. *Curr Opinion Urol* **8**, 5–9.

Trucchi A, Tubaro A, Romano & Carter SS (1998). Ultrasound imaging of the prostate in patients with lower urinary tract symptoms. *J Endourology* **12**, S156.

Tubaro A, Carter SS, de-la-Rosette J, Hofner K, Trucchi A, Ogden C, Miano L, Valenti M, Jonas U & Debruyne F (1995). The prediction of clinical outcome from transurethral microwave thermotherapy by pressure-flow analysis: a European multicenter study [see comments]. *J Urol* **153**, 1526–30.

Walker RM, Mamczasz H, Romano G & Carter SS (1997a). Cost effectiveness of routine pressure-flow studies in men with lower urinary tract symptoms. *Br J Urol* **79** (Suppl.), 17.

Walker RM, Romano G, Tubaro A, Davies A, Theodoreou N, Springall R & Carter SS (1997b). The results of pressure flow studies in a control population of male patients greater than 45 years. *Br J Urol* **70**(Suppl.), 17.

Walker RM, Patel A & St Clair Carter S (1998). Is there a clinically significant change in pressure-flow study values after urethral instrumentation in patients with lower urinary tract symptoms? *Br J Urol* **81**, 206–10.

Witjes WP, Aarnink RG, Ezz-el-Din K, Wijkstra H, Debruyne EM & de la Rosette JJ (1997). The correlation between prostate volume, transition zone volume, transition zone index and clinical and urodynamic investigations in patients with lower urinary tract symptoms. *Br J Urol* **80**, 84–90.

Chapter 4

Effective differential diagnosis: excluding prostate cancer

John Anderson

Introduction

At first sight it may seem perverse to discuss prostate cancer in a book on benign prostate enlargement (BPE). Bladder outflow obstruction and prostate cancer are both equally important health issues, but what is their connection?

Altered patterns of micturition are common in older men and cause concern about the nature of any underlying disease in the prostate. With increasing awareness of health issues in general and media attention on prostate cancer in particular, the spectre of malignant disease is raised in the mind of many such patients. BPE is also an increasing problem with advancing years and although there is no evidence to suggest a causal association with cancer of the prostate, both conditions occur in men of a similar age. Thus the fear of prostate cancer may be the main reason for a patient to consult his doctor in the first instance. Once he can be reassured that there is no evidence of malignancy, he can cope with the mild urinary symptoms which are often of no more than nuisance value.

From the other viewpoint, the doctor or clinical nurse practitioner must be alert to a possible diagnosis of prostate cancer during the routine investigation of men with lower urinary tract symptoms (LUTS). There are justified concerns regarding either an unsuspected diagnosis of prostate cancer in such men, or worse still, missing that diagnosis. To fail to detect an early prostate cancer in an elderly unfit man is probably less important than the benefits gained by identifying the disease at an early stage in someone who is younger and fitter when potentially 'curative' treatment is available. To this end, I will outline a rationale as to why I believe it is important to look for prostate cancer in men presenting with LUTS, how we should do this and when it is appropriate.

Facts and figures

Prostate cancer is a major public health issue in the UK. In 1990 the incidence in England and Wales was reported to be 13,481 (54.5 per 100,000 of the male population) (Chamberlain 1997) and it is now the second commonest cause of cancer death in men. The annual mortality rate for prostate cancer has risen by 40 per cent since 1971 and in 1993 there were 8,689 deaths from prostate cancer (Office for National Statistics 1996) – a rate of 33.8 per 100,000. The incidence of the disease has also increased steadily over the last 20 years, due to better identification of cases by cancer registers, improved diagnostic accuracy and increased case finding by measuring serum PSA and histological examination of prostatic tissue removed at the time of surgery for bladder outflow obstruction (BOO).

Until the advent of serum PSA estimation, the majority of patients with prostate cancer presented only once they had become symptomatic with locally advanced or metastatic disease. Not surprisingly, the overall 5-year survival rates in such patients was as low as 36 per cent (Office of Population Censuses and Surveys 1981). It is interesting to compare this figure with the current situation in the USA where early detection programmes and screening allow diagnosis at an earlier stage and where the overall 5-year survival rate is at least 60–70 per cent.

Clearly then, prostate cancer is a common disease where symptoms tend to occur late. If left untreated until this point the tumour will inevitably progress, eventually metastasise and ultimately kill the patient. To make any impact on the course of this disease we need to diagnose prostate cancer at an earlier stage before symptoms develop, and treat it aggressively where appropriate. The case for investigation to detect early asymptomatic prostate cancer in 'prostate clinics' set up to assess BOO would seem self-evident. Furthermore, a proportion of men with more locally advanced prostate cancer will present to such clinics with LUTS and a correct diagnosis is important to allow appropriate treatment.

Before considering the techniques and value of investigation for prostate cancer in this setting, it is worthwhile considering the natural history of prostate cancer and how this may have a bearing on the patient's presentation, particularly in the context of patients being investigated for LUTS. It is important to distinguish three types of prostate cancer:

- 'latent' or incidental prostate cancer
- early or clinically localised significant disease
- locally advanced or metastatic disease.

The clinical significance of latent prostate cancer is unclear and there is no natural progression from this microscopic diagnosis to clinically significant malignancy, although there is a natural progression from localised disease to more locally advanced and then metastatic disease as a function of time.

'Latent' or incidental prostate cancer

The high incidence of microscopic foci of well-differentiated cancer detected in the prostate at autopsy studies has long been recognised (Franks 1954). The prevalence rates increase with age but are acknowledged to be insignificant as a cause of death (Whittemore *et al.* 1991). Unlike clinically detectable tumours, which are more common in the industrialised Western world, there is a similar worldwide geographical distribution of latent prostate cancer (Yatani *et al.* 1982) suggesting that some form of 'activation' of this disease process by environmental carcinogens is required to produce a clinically significant cancer. Latent or incidental prostate cancers typically have a volume of <0.2 ml and are too small to feel, too small to cause an elevation of the serum prostate-specific antigen (PSA) and invisible on transrectal ultrasound scanning (TRUS) (McNeal *et al.* 1986). It is very unlikely that these clinically insignificant tumours will be identified during routine investigation in a prostate assessment clinic.

Early or localised prostate cancer

A clinically significant early prostate cancer is one which occupies a volume of >0.5 ml (Stamey *et al.* 1993). Such tumours rarely produce symptoms and are detected by digital rectal examination (DRE), an elevated serum PSA, or on TRUS with systematic sextant biopsies of the prostate. Untreated, they will increase in size with time, extend locally and eventually metastasise to the regional lymphatics or to bone. To diagnose such a tumour while it is still confined to the prostate, particularly in younger men where definitive potentially curative treatment is still available, is one of the main benefits of any form of 'prostatic screening clinic'.

While evaluation of LUTS is the main purpose of prostate assessment clinics, early detection of localised prostate cancer in young fit men is undoubtedly an additional bonus.

Locally advanced or metastatic prostate cancer

Many patients with local spread of cancer beyond the prostate present with LUTS and a correct diagnosis is essential if appropriate treatment is to be instituted. Such tumours are usually easily palpable on DRE and cause an elevation of the serum PSA. Unsuspected metastatic disease may be identified on a bone scan or the patient may complain of bone pain (typically progressive back pain due to secondaries in the pelvic bones and lumbar spine) or systemic symptoms such as lethargy (due to anaemia resulting from bone marrow involvement), weight loss and cachexia. While such patients will derive significant symptomatic benefit from hormone manipulation, to treat their LUTS in isolation is less than ideal.

There are three important questions which need to be addressed when considering effective differential diagnosis in the prostate clinic, and particularly in the diagnosis of prostate cancer:

- Are there effective tests to help us make the diagnosis?
- Having diagnosed prostate cancer, is there effective treatment for the disease?
- Do early diagnosis and aggressive treatment improve the long-term outcome?

How do we diagnose prostate cancer?

The diagnosis of prostate cancer depends on a digital rectal examination (DRE), estimation of the serum PSA and TRUS with systemic sextant biopsies whenever either is abnormal.

DRE is part of the routine examination of any patient with LUTS, both to make some estimate of the size of the gland and to exclude features suggestive of malignancy. An overtly malignant-feeling gland with a locally advanced tumour typically feels 'stony' hard in one or both lobes of the prostate, quite unlike the normal consistency of the prostate which is likened to the feel of the flesh over the palmar aspect of the head of the fifth metacarpal. (Malignancy feels like the flesh over the dorsal aspect of the head of the fifth metacarpal). A less obvious tumour may provide a feeling of induration in either lobe of the prostate, but in true early or localised cancer the tumour may be completely impalpable.

PSA is an enzyme produced almost exclusively by the prostate. It is normally secreted into the prostatic fluid but is also detectable in the serum. Any abnormality in the prostate is sufficient to cause an elevation in the serum levels of the PSA. It is important to recognise that PSA is specific for the prostate, not for cancer, and an elevated PSA may commonly be due to benign prostatic enlargement, prostatitis or manipulation of the prostate, as well as an early cancer. It has been estimated that 1 g of benign prostatic hyperplasia (BPH) will raise the PSA by 0.3 ng/ml, while 1 g of cancer will raise it higher by an extra factor of 10 at 3.5 ng/ml (McNeal *et al.* 1986). Since BPH is more prevalent than cancer, the commonest cause of a marginally elevated PSA is benign prostatic enlargement. Inevitably then, there is a grey area where a slight elevation of the serum PSA may be due to either BPH or cancer.

The concept of a 'normal' PSA is inappropriate and the 'normal' ranges we use reflect these difficulties. In an attempt to define a normal PSA Catalona *et al.* (1991) invited asymptomatic men over the age of 50 for prostate cancer 'screening'. It was agreed that if their serum PSA was greater than 4 ng/ml, they would undergo transrectal ultrasound screening and prostate biopsy. In all some 1,653 men had their PSA measured and of these 92 per cent were reassured to find their PSA was less than 4 ng/ml. Six per cent (107), however, had a PSA between 4 and 10 ng/ml and, of these, 85 had a biopsy. Nineteen (22 per cent) of them were found to have unsuspected cancer of the prostate. Two per cent (30) had a PSA of more than 10 ng/ml and in those who underwent scans and biopsies the cancer detection rate was 67 per cent. One can see, therefore, that the lower the cut-off for PSA, the more sensitive the test in detecting all cancers, but the less specific for an abnormal level being due to cancer.

Some poorly differentiated prostate cancer may only express PSA in small amounts and therefore the diagnosis may be missed in up to 10 per cent of patients with such tumours if we rely solely on PSA estimation. Combining the serum PSA results with the DRE findings allows such tumours to be detected and therefore routine investigation for prostate cancer necessarily includes both modalities (Catalona *et al.* 1994).

In an attempt to increase the specificity of PSA testing, a number of modifications have been suggested. Since BPE is a function of age, and the PSA is correspondingly raised as men get older, it has been proposed that 'age-specific' ranges of PSA may more reliably differentiate those with elevated PSA due to prostate cancer (Oesterling 1996). This will inevitably make the PSA test more sensitive in young men in whom early diagnosis can be important, and more specific in the elderly who need to avoid unnecessary biopsies.

To minimise the risk of an elevated PSA being simply due to BPE, others have suggested correlating the serum PSA to the volume of the prostate as measured at TRUS to produce a figure for the PSA density (PSAD) (Benson *et al.* 1992). If the PSAD is less than 0.15, the chance of the raised PSA being due to cancer is increased. To obtain this figure, however, one needs to carry out a TRUS and it would seem far more appropriate to biopsy the prostate at that stage rather than depend on an unreliable mathematical calculation.

If there is an underlying cancer in the prostate, one would expect the PSA to rise progressively more quickly than in simple BPE. This rate of change of the PSA or PSA velocity (PSAV) (Smith & Catalona 1994) has been used to predict an underlying cancer where biopsy has been deferred after the initial estimation and where there is concern. The possibility of metastases is increased once the PSA increases by more than 0.75 ng/ml/year, although again this is not absolute.

Recent developments have shown that PSA is expressed in a number of molecular forms with the greater part bound to protein, leaving a free fraction of PSA within the serum. The lower the percentage of free unbound PSA in the serum, the greater the chance of underlying prostate cancer, particularly when the figure is less than 15 per cent (Oesterling *et al.* 1995).

The routine use of PSA estimation in prostate assessment clinics is somewhat controversial and given the lack of specificity of a raised PSA for cancer, some information on PSA testing should be given to patients in advance. Counselling should include information about the sensitivity and specificity of PSA levels, on the nature, reliability and complications of prostate biopsy, as well as the uncertainty about the management of prostate cancer. When fully informed of the issues, a man's attitude to PSA testing may change.

If the PSA is elevated or the DRE is suspicious, the patient requires a TRUS and systemic sextant biopsies (Sanders & El Galley 1997). While the sonographic appearances are non-specific for cancer, the best chances of confirming a diagnosis of prostate cancer in a palpably normal gland lie with this type of guided sampling of the prostate.

Objections have been raised to investigation for early prostate cancer in an asymptomatic population and particularly in those who simply present with LUTS to prostate assessment clinics. The point is made that randomised controlled trials have not demonstrated the value of this intervention. Currently, a large European multi-centre randomised trial assessing the value of screening for early prostate cancer is under way (Schroder & Bangma 1997) and recent results from a Canadian study would suggest that screening is effective in reducing the mortality rate for prostate cancer (Labrie *et al.* 1998). Absence of conclusive results from studies does not mean that investigation is not worthwhile. Others would claim that having diagnosed prostate cancer at an early stage the ideal treatment or outcome is not clear. Again, this does not mean that we should avoid early diagnosis and in the next section we will examine the evidence for effective treatment for early prostate cancer.

Is there effective treatment for early prostate cancer?

Treatment for early prostate cancer ranges from nothing, or more correctly, 'watchful waiting' until the disease progresses, to radical radiotherapy or radical surgery. At first sight one might suspect that intervention has little to offer if doing nothing is a real option. However, it is important to recognise that prostate cancer may present at different ages in patients with different co-morbidity and therefore different life expectancy, to understand how each of these treatment options may have their own merits as well as disadvantages.

The case for watchful waiting is most strongly represented by the Scandinavian experience. Johanssen *et al.* (1997) reported in a study of 642 men with prostate cancer that only 11 per cent of 300 with localised disease died of the disease. As with many such studies these results need interpretation. The mean age of all patients in this study was 72 years with 15 per cent of men older than 80 years. The large majority (81 per cent) had well- or moderately differentiated tumours, with 84 per cent of cases being diagnosed by fine-needle aspiration cytology, a technique with a high false positive rate. Furthermore, the impact of tumour stage and grade and age on survival rates is not specified. It would seem reasonable to conclude that expectant treatment in elderly men with low-grade, low-stage prostatic cancer and associated co-morbidity limiting their long-term life expectancy is a reasonable option. This is certainly not the case for a fit 50-year-old man with early prostate cancer. The results from a pooled analysis of six large series of patients treated by watchful waiting show that a man with a moderately differentiated tumour has a 52 per cent chance of developing metastatic disease within ten years (Chodak *et al.* 1994). The case for active intervention in younger fitter men with a life expectancy of more than ten years would seem clear-cut.

If a cancer is truly confined to the prostate with no evidence of extraprostatic spread, one can understand how total removal of the prostate may provide potential 'cure' from the disease. Excellent long-term results have been obtained using this technique. In a pooled analysis of 2,758 radical prostatectomies performed on men with clinically localised prostate cancer, ten-year metastasis-free survival was up to 68 per cent for moderately and 52 per cent for poorly differentiated tumours (Gerber *et al.* 1996). Radical surgery is not without its problems, however. The overall mortality rate is up to 1 per cent, complete incontinence can occur in around 5 per cent and impotence in at least two-thirds of patients (Murphy *et al.* 1994). Despite these disadvantages, quality of life studies show a minimal effect and up to 89 per cent of patients would undergo the procedure again if necessary, knowing their diagnosis (Fowler *et al.* 1995).

Given the disparity of the treatment options for such a common disease, it is perhaps surprising that randomised controlled trials have not demonstrated superiority for one form of treatment over another. Attempts to address this question by the Medical Research Council in the UK failed when it proved impossible to recruit patients to a randomised trial of watchful waiting versus surgery versus radiotherapy. While patients agreed that such a trial was the right way to answer the question, they were reluctant to have treatment for their own cancer decided at random and the trial closed after three years having recruited only 35 of an intended 1,800 patients (MRC Working Party on Prostate Cancer 1996). Ongoing studies in the USA have similar recruitment problems but a smaller Scandinavian study will provide useful information, albeit having excluded poorly differentiated cancers.

While the relative effectiveness of the three main treatment options is still not known, the clinician is left with a dilemma as to how to manage patients with newly diagnosed early prostate cancer. 'Watchful waiting', because of its lower incidence of side-effects, would seem to be the best option for men with less than ten years' life expectancy, especially those with low-volume well-differentiated tumours. Active intervention, particularly with radical surgery, can provide potential 'cure' for younger fitter men with results equivalent to a normal life expectancy. The morbidity of the procedure can be minimised in the hands of 'sub-specialists', and patients and their families are often prepared to accept more morbidity in a trade-off for (assumed) survival benefit (Litwin *et al.* 1995).

Do early detection and treatment make a difference?

Effective early diagnosis and treatment for prostate cancer should result in earlier stage disease at diagnosis and improved survival rates for prostate cancer. It should not increase the diagnosis of clinically insignificant cancers, with attendant anxiety and possibly unnecessary treatment. Such evidence is hard to come by in the UK but data now coming out of the USA, where a more aggressive approach to the diagnosis and treatment of prostate cancer is taken, would suggest that early detection programmes can achieve these desired aims.

The National Cancer Institute's Surveillance, Epidemiology and End Results (SEER) programme consists of nine regional tumour registries that abstract information from medical records on all cancer diagnosed within their defined geographic areas. These large population studies allow changing trends in incidence, stage at presentation, treatment and survival rates to be analysed from 1973.

Figure 4.1 shows that the incidence of prostate cancer in the Seattle-Puget Sound region increased slowly from 1974 to 1984 (Newcomer *et al.* 1997). Thereafter the

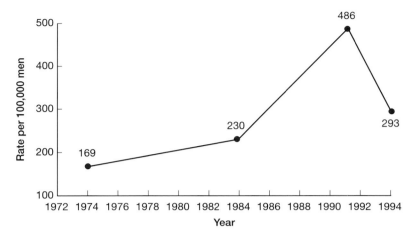

Figure 4.1 Prostate cancer incidence in Western Washington State, 1974–94

dramatic rise and subsequent fall in incident prostate cancer cases was unprecedented in cancer surveillance. The timing of these changes paralleled the introduction of PSA screening. As incident cases are identified and withdrawn from the potential pool of new diagnoses, eventually the incidence will fall. The data here suggest that this has occurred and certainly PSA testing does not appear to be going on to detect increasing numbers of clinically insignificant latent cancers. Interestingly, all stages of prostate cancer followed the same incidence trend peaking in 1991, except metastatic disease, which peaked in 1986 and subsequently declined by over 60 per cent, from 42/100,000 to 18/100,000 in 1994.

Commensurate with this increasing incidence of prostate cancer but decreasing proportion of advanced disease, the radical prostatectomy rate in the USA has risen from 9.2 per cent of all prostate cancer patients in 1974 to 29 per cent of all newly diagnosed cases in 1993 (Mettlin *et al.* 1997). Not only is the disease being picked up more frequently and at an earlier stage, but active treatment has followed early diagnosis. The final part of the jigsaw appears to have fallen into place when for the first time the overall mortality rate from prostate cancer fell for the first time, from 26.5/100,000 in 1990 to 17.3/100,000 men in 1995 (SEER Programme 1997). While it would seem relatively early for this result to follow on from early detection programmes and the widespread use of PSA testing, the results are unexpected and difficult to interpret in any other way.

Conclusions

The potential to screen for early prostate cancer in prostate assessment clinics should be viewed as a bonus. To detect a clinically significant prostate cancer while it is still confined to the prostate gland in a fit young man when it is still potentially curable should be considered as a definite advantage. To fail to detect a small tumour in an elderly unfit man with associated co-morbidity is not of great clinical relevance to the patient as a whole, and should not deter early detection in those who may benefit from an early diagnosis. To identify a more locally advanced tumour in a man with LUTS is equally important to ensure that appropriate treatment is started for the cancer and not just symptomatic treatment for outflow obstruction.

To maximise these benefits for prostate assessment clinics the algorithm in Figure 4.2 provides an appropriate set of guidelines to follow. All patients should have a DRE. If the DRE is abnormal or the patient is concerned, the serum PSA level should be measured. If the rectal examination is normal, the patient is less than 70 years old and otherwise fit, a PSA estimation is indicated after appropriate explanation as to the limitations of the test. If the serum PSA is <4 ng/ml, the patient can be reasonably assured that the risk of cancer is minimal, although annual PSA estimations thereafter may be appropriate. If the PSA is >10 ng/ml, the chance of cancer being present outweighs any other cause for an elevated PSA, and TRUS and systematic sextant biopsies are indicated. If these fail to confirm the diagnosis, a repeat PSA in three or six months' time and possible further biopsies are advisable. For those with a serum PSA in the equivocal grey area of 4–10 ng/ml a low percentage free PSA may help direct the decision to TRUS and biopsy at this stage. Alternatively, a full discussion with the patient about the risks of cancer (around 25 per cent) may allow him to pursue active investigation at that stage or await the results of a repeat PSA in three or six months' time.

In the face of a normal DRE, men over 70, or who are otherwise unfit, do not require routine PSA estimation.

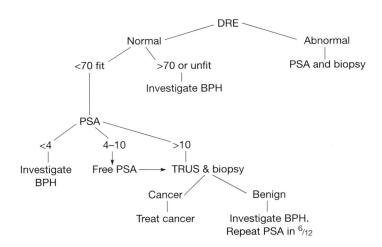

Figure 4.2 Effective differential diagnosis to detect prostate cancer in prostate assessment clinics

References

Benson MC, Ehang IS, Pantuck A *et al.* (1992). Prostate specific antigen density: a means of distinguishing benign prostatic hypertrophy and prostate cancer. *J Urol* **147**, 813–21.

Catalona WJ, Smith DS, Ratliff TL *et al.* (1991). Measurement of prostate specific antigen in serum as a screening test for prostate cancer. *N Eng J Med* **324**, 1156–61.

Catalona WJ, Richie JP, Ahmann FR *et al.* (1994). Comparision of digital rectal examination and serum prostate specific antigen in the early detection of prostate cancer: results of a multicentre clinical trial of 6630 men. *J Urol* **151**, 1283–90.

Chamberlain J, Melia J, Moss J & Brown J (1997). Report prepared for the health technology assessment panel of the NHS Executive on the diagnosis, management, treatment and costs of prostate cancer in England and Wales. *B J Urol* **79**(Suppl. 3), 1–32.

Chodak GW, Thisted RA, Gerber GS *et al.* (1994). Results of conservative management of clinically localised prostate cancer. *N Eng J Med* **330**, 242–8.

Fowler FJ, Wasson J, Barry MJ, Roman A, Lu-Yao G & Wennberg J (1995). Effect of radical prostatectomy for prostate cancer on patient quality of life; results from a Medicare survey. *Urology* **45**, 1007–15.

Franks LM (1954). Latent carcinoma of the prostate. *J Pathol Bacteriol* **68**, 603–16.

Gerber GS, Thisted RA, Scardino PT *et al.* (1996). Results of radical prostatectomy in men with clinically localised prostate cancer. *JAMA* **276**, 615–19.

Johanssen JE, Holmberg L, Johansson S, Bergstrom R & Admani HO (1997). Fifteen year survival in prostate cancer. A prospective population-based study in Sweden. *JAMA* **277**, 467.

Labrie F, Dupont A, Candas B *et al.* (1998). Decrease of prostate cancer deaths by screening: first data from the Quebec prospective and randomised study. *Proc ASCO* **17**, 4.

Litwin MS, Hays RD, Fink A *et al.* (1995). Quality of life outcomes in men treated for localised prostate cancer. *JAMA* **273**, 129–35.

McNeal JE, Kindrachuk RA, Freiha FS, Bostwick DG, Redwine EA & Stamey TA (1986). Patterns of progression in prostate cancer. *Lancet* **1**, 60–3.

MRC Working Party on Prostate Cancer (1996). Total prostatectomy, radiotherapy or no immediate treatment for early prostate cancer. A randomised trial (PRO6). MRC Cancer Trials Office, Cambridge.

Mettlin C, Murphy GP & Menck HR (1997). Changes in patterns of prostate care in the United States: results of American College of Surgeons Commission on Cancer Studies, 1974–93. *Prostate* **32**, 221–6.

Murphy GP, Mettlin C, Menck H, Winchester DP & Davidson M (1994). National patterns of prostate cancer treatment by radical prostatectomy: results of a survey by the American College of Surgeons Commission on Cancer. *J Urol* **152**, 1817–19.

Newcomer LM, Stanford JL, Blumenstein BA & Brawer MK (1997). Temporal trends in rates of prostatic cancer: declining incidence of advanced stage disease, 1974–1994. *J Urol* **158**, 1427–30.

Oesterling JE (1996). Age specific reference ranges for serum PSA. *N Eng J Med* **335**, 345–6.

Oesterling JE, Jacobsen SJ, Klee GG *et al.* (1995). Free, complexed and total serum prostate specific antigen: the establishment of appropriate reference ranges for their concentrations and ratios. *J Urol* **154**, 1090–5.

Office for National Statistics (1996). *Mortality statistics: cause. England and Wales. 1993 (revised) and 1994.* Series DH2, No. 21. HMSO, London.

Office of Population Censuses and Surveys (1981). *Cancer statistics. Incidence, survival and mortality in England and Wales.* No. 43. HMSO, London.

Sanders H & El Galley R (1997). Ultrasound findings are not useful for defining stage IIc prostate cancer. *World J Urol* **15**, 336–8.

Schroder FH & Bangma CH (1997). European randomised trial of screening (ERSPC). *Br J Urol* **79**(Suppl.), 68–71.

Smith DS & Catalona WJ (1994). Rate of change in serum prostate specific antigen levels as a method for prostate cancer detection. *J Urol* **152**, 1163–7.

Stamey TA, Freiha FS, McNeal JE *et al.* (1993). Localised prostate cancer: relationship of tumour volume to clinical significance for the treatment of prostate cancer. *Cancer* **71**, 933–8.

Surveillance, Epidemiology and End Results (SEER) Programme (1997). Age adjusted US cancer death rates. *J Natl Cancer Inst* **89**, 12.

Whittemore AS, Keller AB & Betensky R (1991). Low grade, latent prostate cancer volume: predictor of clinical cancer incidence? *J Natl Cancer Inst* **83**, 1231–5.

Yatani R, Chigusa I, Akazaki K, Stemmerman GN, Welsh RA & Correa P (1982). Geographic pathology of latent prostatic carcinoma. *Int J Cancer* **29**, 611–61.

PART 2

Evidence and treatment

Chapter 5

The evidence-base for medical intervention

Richard Bell and Paul Abrams

Introduction

Histological benign prostatic hyperplasia (BPH) is one of the most common disease processes affecting older men; autopsy studies show an increasing incidence of BPH with age, from approximately 10 per cent in 40-year-old men to almost 90 per cent in men over the age of 80 years (Moore RA 1943; Berry *et al.* 1984). The variation in age-specific prevalence of histological BPH in different populations is very small (Bostwick *et al.* 1992), but the extent to which it leads to benign prostatic enlargement (BPE) with lower urinary tract symptoms (LUTS) and benign prostatic obstruction (BPO) is significant. The reported prevalence of LUTS suggestive of BPO in older men in community-based studies varies between 17 and 50 per cent (Jensen *et al.* 1986; Garraway *et al.* 1991; Diokno *et al.* 1992; Chute *et al.* 1993; Wolfs *et al.* 1994; Tsukamoto *et al.* 1995; Trueman *et al.* 1999), with approximately 1 in 4 men receiving treatment for this in the eighth decade of life (Jacobsen *et al.* 1999). Health-related quality of life appears to be reduced in men with benign prostatic enlargement (Girman *et al.* 1999).

Transurethral resection of the prostate (TURP) remains the gold standard treatment for BPO, with approximately 28,000 performed annually in the UK (Office of Population Censuses and Surveys 1985). However, it is a procedure not without risks (Mebust *et al.* 1989; Doll *et al.* 1992), and concerns over increased long-term cardiovascular morbidity following TURP have not been resolved (Roos *et al.* 1989; Malenka *et al.* 1990; Fugslig *et al.* 1994). LUTS, however, have a poor diagnostic specificity for bladder outlet obstruction (BOO) (Neal *et al.* 1989), and approximately 20 per cent of patients have persistent LUTS following TURP (Ezz el Din *et al.* 1996). The eight-year re-operation rate following TURP is significant (Roos *et al.* 1989). The natural history of BPO is such that 40–56 per cent of patients will achieve a spontaneous improvement in their LUTS with just watchful waiting (Craigen *et al.* 1969; Ball *et al.* 1981; Kadow *et al.* 1988; Wasson *et al.* 1995).

Clearly, there is a group of patients where refractory urinary retention, obstructive uropathy, associated bladder calculi and recurrent urinary tract infections are indications for surgical intervention. However, a significant number of men without these indications have moderate symptoms (American Urological Association Symptom Score 8–18) that are not sufficiently bothersome to warrant surgical intervention, but who do not wish to be managed by watchful waiting (McConnell *et al.* 1994). It is this group of patients that is ideally suited to a trial of medical therapy. Patients unfit for, or awaiting TURP, may also be considered for medical treatment.

The current options available for the medical treatment of BPO include:

- α-adrenoceptor antagonists
- endocrine treatment
- phytotherapy.

α-adrenoceptor antagonists

The pathophysiological basis of α-blockade

The presence and contractile response of α-adrenoceptors within the bladder neck, prostatic adenoma and capsule have been described by Caine *et al.* (1975b). Although both α_1- and α_2-adrenoceptors are present within the prostatic stroma (Lepor & Shapiro 1984), it is the α_1-adrenoceptors that are responsible for prostatic urethral tone (Hedlund *et al.* 1985; Shapiro & Lepor 1986; Kitada & Kumazawa 1987; Chapple *et al.* 1989), contributing approximately 40 per cent of total urethral pressure in patients with BPO (Furuya *et al.* 1982). There also appears to be an increase in stromal density of α_1-adrenoceptors in hyperplastic prostatic tissue (Yamada *et al.* 1987; Chapple *et al.* 1989; Nasu *et al.* 1996).

Pharmacological and receptor cloning studies have identified at least three α_1-adrenoceptor subtypes. Recently, consensus over nomenclature has been reached (Hieble *et al.* 1995). The native subtypes of α_1-adrenoceptors are designated α_{1A}, α_{1B} and α_{1D} (corresponding to previous cloned subtypes alpha-1c, alpha-1b and alpha-1a/d respectively). The respective cloned counterparts are differentiated by lower case letters (α_{1a}, α_{1b} and α_{1d}). All three subtypes have been demonstrated within the prostate (Andersson *et al.* 1997), with the α_{1a} subtype being the most prevalent (Nasu *et al.* 1996). Expression of the three receptor subtypes appears to be altered in BPH, with a reduction expression of α_{1B} receptors (Walden *et al.* 1999). Studies by Forray *et al.* (1994) and Marshall *et al.* (1995) suggest that it is the α_{1A}-adrenoceptor subtype that effects the contractile response of the prostatic smooth muscle to noradrenaline. However, α_1-adrenoceptors within the prostate can also be divided on the basis of affinity to prazosin – those with high affinity (α_{1H}) and those with low affinity (α_{1L}) (Muramatsu *et al.* 1994). A possible role for the α_{1L} receptor in the contractile response of the prostate has been proposed (Ford *et al.* 1996; Kenny *et al.* 1996). Thus although there appears to be good evidence for the role of α_1-adrenoceptors in the contractile response of the prostate, there is no consensus regarding the exact subtype of α_1-adrenoceptor responsible.

Both doxazosin and terazosin appear to induce stromal and epithelial cell apoptosis, and a parallel reduction in smooth muscle cells, which correlates with the improvement in LUTS (Chon *et al.* 1999).

Historical studies

Initial studies using α-adrenergic blockers in patients with BPO were with the combined α_1- and α_2-adrenergic antagonists phenoxybenzamine and phentolamine (Caine *et al.* 1976; Whitfield *et al.* 1976; Caine *et al.* 1978). These confirmed a significant improvement in LUTS, with increased maximum and mean flow rates and a decrease in urethral closure pressure with combined α-blockade, but at the expense of a significant side-effect profile (Caine *et al.* 1978, 1981; Abrams *et al.* 1982), with up to 29 per cent of patients experiencing dizziness (Abrams *et al.* 1982). Inhibition of the presynaptic α_2-adrenergic receptors with subsequent impairment of synaptic re-uptake of noradrenaline is the proposed mechanism for many of the side-effects observed with combined α-blockade. Subsequent studies on the use of α-blockers in BPO have concentrated on α_1-specific adrenoceptor antagonists in an attempt to reduce unwanted side-effects while maintaining efficacy.

The placebo effect

It is apparent from 'watchful waiting' studies that there is a significant variability in the natural history of LUTS suggestive of BPO, with 40–56 per cent of men improving spontaneously (Craigen *et al.* 1969; Ball *et al.* 1981; Kadow *et al.* 1988; Wasson *et al.* 1995). Against this background rate of spontaneous improvement it is evident that any novel therapy for the treatment of BPO must be compared to a placebo or sham treatment (Cockett *et al.* 1993). Analysis of 45 placebo-controlled trials of medical therapy for BPO reveals approximately a 40 per cent mean symptom improvement with placebo alone (McConnell *et al.* 1994).

Selective α_1-adrenoceptor antagonists in current use

The inhibitory action of the α_1-specific adrenoceptor (α_1-AR) antagonists on human prostatic tissue *in vitro* was confirmed with prazosin (Shapiro *et al.* 1981). The efficacy of prazosin in the treatment of BPO was later confirmed in placebo-controlled trials (Hedlund *et al.* 1983; Kirby *et al.* 1987; Chapple *et al.* 1990). Subsequently, the efficacy of other α_1-AR antagonists – originally designed as anti-hypertensive agents – in men with LUTS suggestive of BPO has been proven in placebo-controlled studies. These include the short-acting indoramin (Chow *et al.* 1990) and alfuzosin (Jardin *et al.* 1991; Buzelin *et al.* 1993, 1996), and the long-acting terazosin (Lepor *et al.* 1992; Brawer *et al.* 1993; Roehrborn *et al.* 1996; Elhilali *et al.* 1996; Lepor *et al.* 1996) and doxazosin (Christensen *et al.* 1993; Chapple *et al.* 1994a; Fawzy *et al.* 1995; Gillenwater *et al.* 1995). Tamsulosin – an α_{1A}-subtype-selective adrenoceptor antagonist (Chapple *et al.* 1994b; Minneman *et al.* 1994; Testa *et al.* 1994) specifically designed for the treatment of BPO – has also been extensively investigated in dose-ranging and placebo-controlled trials (Abrams *et al.* 1995; Chapple *et al.* 1996; Lepor & the Tamsulosin Investigator Group 1996; Abrams *et al.* 1997).

These studies have shown a similar efficacy in BPO among the α_1-AR-blockers in common clinical use, with a statistically significant improvement in mean symptom score (14–49 per cent), maximum urinary flow rate (Q_{max}, 13–34 per cent) and average urinary flow rate (Q_{ave}, 11–41 per cent) when compared to placebo (Gillenwater *et al.* 1961; Jardin *et al.* 1991; Lepor *et al.* 1992; Brawer *et al.* 1993; Buzelin *et al.* 1993;

Christensen *et al.* 1993; Chapple *et al.* 1994a, 1994b; Minneman *et al.* 1994; Testa *et al.* 1994; Abrams *et al.* 1995; Fawzy *et al.* 1995; Buzelin *et al.* 1996; Chapple *et al.* 1996; Elhilali *et al.* 1996; Lepor *et al.* 1996; Lepor & the Tamsulosin Investigator Group 1996; Roehrborn *et al.* 1996; Abrams *et al.* 1997; Narayan & Tewari 1998; Michel *et al.* 1998a). However, mean improvements in Q_{max} and Q_{ave} are modest, ranging from 0.7–4.0 ml/s.

Few studies have confirmed a diagnosis of BPO in their study population of men with LUTS using pressure-flow urodynamics. However, the overall prevalence of BOO in men with LUTS is 60 per cent (Reynard *et al.* 1998). Terazosin (Witjes *et al.* 1997), doxazosin (Gerber *et al.* 1996) and tamsulosin (Abrams *et al.* 1997; McNicholas *et al.* 1998) have been shown to produce a significant improvement in pressure-flow urodynamic parameters in patients with documented BPO. However, those patients with LUTS who were not obstructed had equally significant improvements in symptom scores and Q_{max} (Witjes *et al.* 1997; McNicholas *et al.* 1998), suggesting that pressure-flow studies are unnecessary prior to commencement of α-blockers in men with LUTS.

Because of the similarity in efficacy of the available $α_1$-AR antagonists (Djavan & Marberger 1999), comparison between drugs must be based by necessity on pharmacodynamics and side-effect profiles. The modest theoretical advantage of increased compliance with the once-daily dosage (Greenberg 1986) of the long-acting $α_1$-AR antagonists tamsulosin, doxazosin and terazosin has not been confirmed in clinical trials in BPO. Prazosin and terazosin require dose-titration to reduce the 'first-dose phenomenon' of postural hypotension and optimise the efficacy:adverse-event ratio. The beneficial effects of doxazosin on the lipid profile (Neaton *et al.* 1993) and other cardiovascular risk factors in hypertensive patients, the reduction in coronary heart disease (Langdon & Packard 1994) and erectile dysfunction (Neaton *et al.* 1993) make it a treatment choice in hypertensive men with LUTS (Fawzy *et al.* 1999) and those with a history of erectile dysfunction. Both tamsulosin and terazosin, however, appear to be a safe treatment for both normotensive and hypertensive men receiving additional antihypersensitive therapy (Kirby 1998; Michel *et al.* 1998b). The adverse-event profiles of the $α_1$-AR antagonists in common clinical use are well documented (Jardin *et al.* 1991; Lepor *et al.* 1992; Brawer *et al.* 1993; Buzelin *et al.* 1993; Christensen *et al.* 1993; Chapple *et al.* 1994a; Fawzy *et al.* 1995; Buzelin *et al.* 1996; Elhilali *et al.* 1996; Lepor *et al.* 1996; Roehrborn *et al.* 1996) and include dizziness, headache, lethargy, asthenia, postural hypotension and retrograde ejaculation. Terazosin does not appear to affect prostate specific antigen levels (Brawer *et al.* 1999).

Few studies have directly compared the *clinical uroselectivity* (benefit:risk ratio) of different α-blockers. Buzelin *et al.* (1993) described a lower incidence of hypotensive side-effects with alfuzosin compared with prazosin, and a similar adverse-event profile compared with tamsulosin (Buzelin *et al.* 1997). This study together with the similarity of the adverse-event profile of alfuzosin to placebo in other randomised studies (Jardin *et al.* 1991; Buzelin *et al.* 1996) lends some support to claims of alfuzosin's *functional uroselectivity* (Martin *et al.* 1997). The Chinese Tamsulosin Study Group showed a significantly greater improvement in International Prostate Symptom Score (IPSS) and Q_{ave}, and a reduced side effect profile with tamsulosin compared to terazosin (Na *et al.* 1998).

When compared with a placebo, a statistically significant increased incidence of postural hypotension and lethargy with terazosin (Brawer *et al.* 1993; Lowe 1994; Roehrborn *et al.* 1996), of dizziness and asthenia with terazosin (Lowe 1994; Roehrborn *et al.* 1996) and doxazosin (Fulton *et al.* 1995), and of retrograde ejaculation with terazosin (Roehrborn *et al.* 1996) and tamsulosin (Chapple *et al.* 1996; Hofner *et al.* 1999) has been described. However, the differences in side-effects over placebo are small and overall the α_1-AR antagonists show good clinical uroselectivity and are well tolerated, with 1.5–19.7 per cent of patients withdrawing from trials because of side-effects with the α-blocker, compared with a 0–15.2 per cent withdrawal rate for placebo (Jardin *et al.* 1991; Buzelin *et al.* 1993; Chapple *et al.* 1994a; Lowe 1994; Roehrborn *et al.* 1996; Elhilali *et al.* 1996; Lepor *et al.* 1996). However, overall alfuzosin and tamsulosin appear to be better tolerated than doxazosin, terazosin and prazosin (Djavan & Marberger 1999).

Significant symptomatic improvement in LUTS with modest increase in flow rates are seen in 66–93 per cent of men with BPO treated with α_1-AR antagonists (Kawabe *et al.* 1990; Jardin *et al.* 1991; Abrams *et al.* 1995; Roehrborn *et al.* 1996). The response to α-blockers is rapid and appears to be durable over a four-year period (Lepor 1996). α_1-AR antagonists have become established as the first-line medical therapy in LUTS suggestive of BPO (Chapple *et al.* 1988; Lepor *et al.* 1998).

Endocrine therapy

The pathophysiological basis of androgen withdrawal

The growth and development of the prostate are androgen-dependent (Cunha *et al.* 1987). Testicular androgens appear to have at least a permissive role in the development of BPH. Males castrated prior to puberty (Wilson 1980) and those with 5α-reductase deficiency syndrome (Imperato-McGinley *et al.* 1974) do not develop BPH. Androgen receptor density and intraprostatic dihydrotestosterone (DHT) levels remain normal in the ageing prostate despite a decrease in circulating free testosterone (Walsh *et al.* 1983; Robel *et al.* 1985). Growth factor receptors within the prostate appear to be under androgenic control (Traish & Wotiz 1987). Androgen withdrawal with surgical castration or luteinising hormone-releasing hormone (LHRH) analogues produces a 24–58 per cent mean reduction in prostate volume (Schroeder *et al.* 1986; Peters & Walsh 1987; Gabrilove *et al.* 1989; En & Tveter 1994), with a proportionally greater decrease in epithelial, compared with stromal, volume (Peters & Walsh 1987). Similar reductions in prostatic volume are seen with the steroidal androgen receptor antagonist cyproterone acetate (Bosch *et al.* 1989) and the non-steroidal androgen receptor antagonist bicalutamide (En & Tveter 1993). Although significant improvements in symptom score (Peters & Walsh 1987; En & Tveter 1993, 1994) and urodynamic parameters (En & Tveter 1994) have been described with androgen withdrawal and antagonism, their routine use in BPO is precluded by the almost universal occurrence of impotence and hot flushes with the LHRH analogues (Peters & Walsh 1987; Gabrilove *et al.* 1989; En & Tveter 1994), and the high incidence of nipple pain and gynaecomastia with the anti-androgens (Caine *et al.* 1975a; En & Tveter 1994).

5α-reductase inhibitors

Finasteride

Finasteride is a potent reversible inhibitor of type 2 5α-reductase, the enzyme responsible for converting testosterone to DHT within the prostate (Thigpen *et al.* 1993). It suppresses prostatic DHT by approximately 80–90 per cent (McConnell *et al.* 1992; Norman *et al.* 1993) without suppressing plasma testosterone levels (Rittmaster *et al.* 1989), thus theoretically maintaining libido and sexual function. It produces approximately a 30 per cent reduction in prostatic volume in BPE (Stoner & the Finasteride Study Group 1992), by a combination of cellular atrophy and apoptosis (Rittmaster *et al.* 1996).

Large one- and two-year randomised placebo-controlled trials of finasteride 5 mg daily in men with LUTS suggestive of BPO have confirmed significant reductions in median prostatic volume of 19–26 per cent, with an associated modest reduction in mean symptom score and increase in Q_{max} of 2.0–3.9 and 1.3–1.6 respectively (Gormley *et al.* 1992; The Finasteride Study Group 1993; Andersen *et al.* 1995; Nickel *et al.* 1996). A reduction in the pressure-flow urodynamic parameters of obstruction with finasteride has also been described (Kirby *et al.* 1992; Tammela & Kontturi 1993; Schäfer *et al.* 1999). The fall in detrusor pressure at Q_{max} appears to be greatest in men with larger prostates (Abrams *et al.* 1999). Prostate size has been reported to predict outcome with finasteride, with only men with a prostate volume of >40 cc benefiting from treatment (Boyle *et al.* 1996). Men with a baseline prostate-specific antigen (PSA) greater than 1.4 ng/ml appear to have the greatest benefit:risk ratio with finasteride (Bruskewitz *et al.* 1999). The long-term results of finasteride appear to be durable with a gradual but significant increase in mean Q_{max} and symptom score, and decrease in prostatic volume over a four-year period, when compared to placebo (McConnell *et al.* 1998). In this study finasteride also reduced the risk of acute urinary retention and surgical intervention by approximately 50 per cent (McConnell *et al.* 1998). Generally, finasteride is a safe, well-tolerated drug (Gormley *et al.* 1992; The Finasteride Study Group 1993; Andersen *et al.* 1995; Moore E *et al.* 1995; Boyle *et al.* 1996; Nickel *et al.* 1996; McConnell *et al.* 1998; Hudson *et al.* 1999). Unexpectedly, side-effects are largely related to sexual dysfunction. A small but statistically significant increase in impotence (3.7–15.8 per cent), reduced libido (3.3–6.4 per cent), abnormal ejaculation (2.6–7.7 per cent), gynaecomastia (1.8 per cent) and mastalgia (0.7 per cent) compared to placebo has been described with finasteride

(Gormley *et al.* 1992; The Finasteride Study Group 1993; Nickel *et al.* 1996; McConnell *et al.* 1998). Adverse effects do not appear to increase over time (McConnell *et al.* 1998), and have not led to large numbers of patients discontinuing treatment (Gormley *et al.* 1992; The Finasteride Study Group 1993; Nickel *et al.* 1996; McConnell *et al.* 1998). Treatment failure appears to be uncommon with finasteride, with less than 10 per cent of patients withdrawing from studies for this reason (Gormley *et al.* 1992; The Finasteride Study Group 1993; Stoner & the Finasteride Study Group 1994b; McConnell *et al.* 1998). An improvement in health-related quality of life in men taking finasteride has been described (Byrnes *et al.* 1995; Bruskewitz *et al.* 1999).

Treatment with finasteride may be more cost effective than watchful waiting or α blocker therapy using terazosin (Albertsen *et al.* 1999). The serum PSA level in men with BPE taking finasteride for at least 12 months is reduced by 50 per cent (Guess *et al.* 1993; Stoner & the Finasteride Study Group 1994a). A reduction in PSA is also seen in prostate cancer (Andriole *et al.* 1995). Although the absence of an increased PSA velocity in men on finasteride subsequently found to have prostate cancer has been described (Stoner & the Finasteride Study Group 1994a), to date there is no evidence from long-term studies that finasteride masks prostate cancer (Stoner & the Finasteride Study Group 1994b; McConnell *et al.* 1998; Yang *et al.* 1999). Brawer *et al.* (1999) suggested the heterogeneity of the PSA response to finasteride may make monitoring of patients for the development of prostate cancer problematic. However, the usefulness of PSA in detecting prostate cancer in the PLESS study was maintained by multiplying the total PSA by two (Andriole *et al.* 1998). Free PSA levels do not appear to be altered significantly (Pannek *et al.* 1998).

In men with BPE and LUTS, finasteride appears to be a safe and effective therapy, reducing the complications associated with BPO.

Finasteride and α-blocker combination therapy

The differing modes of action of finasteride and α-blockers should theoretically produce an additive effect when used in combination. A randomised placebo-controlled study in 1,229 men with presumed BPO over one year, comparing terazosin with finasteride or a combination of both drugs, was carried out by Lepor *et al.* (1996). No significant improvement in symptom score or Q_{max} was seen with combination therapy compared with terazosin alone. In contrast to all other studies, no significant difference in symptom score or flow rates was seen with finasteride compared with placebo. A possible reason for this is the smaller mean prostate volume in this study compared with other studies (Kirby *et al.* 1992). However, the lack of any additional benefit in symptom score and Q_{max} with a combination of finasteride and sustained-release alfuzosin compared to sustained-release alfuzosin alone (Debruyne *et al.* 1998) provides further clinical evidence against the use of combination therapy. However, the role of combination therapy in men with LUTS and prostate volumes >40 cc has not been clarified.

Epristeride

Epristeride is an *un*competitive steroidal 5α-reductase types 1 and 2 inhibitor. It has a theoretical advantage over finasteride – a competitive inhibitor of type 2 5α-reductase – in that androgen receptor antagonism should not be affected by the inevitable intraprostatic accumulation of testosterone that occurs with 5α-reductase inhibition. A phase II placebo-controlled study has shown a 74 per cent mean reduction in intraprostatic DHT with epristeride 80 mg daily, without any significant fall in serum testosterone. It appears to be well tolerated at this dose (Peeling *et al.* 1992). Results of phase III studies are awaited.

Oestrogen withdrawal

The role of oestrogens in BPH is less well defined. In the canine prostate BPH model, oestrogens appear to act synergistically with androgens leading to induction of androgen receptors (Walsh & Wilson 1976; Moore RJ *et al.* 1979; Barrack & Berry 1987). In the ageing man there is a relative increase in oestrogen levels compared to testosterone, and intraprostatic levels of oestrogen are higher in those with BPE (Henderson *et al.* 1987). Oestrogens in men are derived mainly from the peripheral aromatisation of testosterone and androstenedione to oestradiol and oestrone respectively. Aromatase enzyme activity in the prostate is greatest within the periurethral zone (Stone *et al.* 1986), which together with the transition zone forms the site of origin of BPH (McNeal 1978). Aromatase inhibition has formed the basis of oestrogen withdrawal trials in BPO.

The aromatase inhibitor testolactone was reported to produce some prostatic shrinkage in an uncontrolled study of 13 men with BPE (Tunn & Schweikurt 1989). However, two randomised placebo-controlled trials of the more potent aromatase inhibitor atamestane failed to show any reduction in prostatic volume or improvement in symptom score and flow rate when compared with placebo, despite significant reductions in serum oestrogen levels (Gingell *et al.* 1995; Radlmaier *et al.* 1996).

Mepartricin (Ipertrofan) is a semisynthetic polyene. It is not absorbed orally, binding to enteric oestrogen thus preventing its enterohepatic recirculation in bile. It significantly reduces serum oestrogen levels in men with BPH (Lotti *et al.* 1988). One randomised placebo-controlled trial of mepartricin 40 mg daily for six months in BPO reported a significant improvement in mean symptom score, Q_{max} and quality of life compared to placebo (Denis *et al.* 1997).

Phytotherapy

There are many different plant extract preparations available for the treatment of LUTS suggestive of BPO. For many of these the mechanism of action is unknown, and their efficacy remains untested in randomised placebo-controlled trials. The few preparations that have been formally assessed are critically reviewed here.

Serenoa repens

Serenoa repens (*Sabal serrulata*) is an extract of the berries from the dwarf palm tree saw palmetto. It is one of the most popular phytotherapeutic agents used in the treatment of BPO, with numerous different preparations available. The active component of the extract is unknown, and the mechanism of action controversial. Of the available preparations, Permixon – a hexane extract of *Serenoa repens* – is the most widely studied. The proposed actions of Permixon include type 1 and 2 5α-reductase inhibitor activity (Di Silverio *et al.* 1996; Bayne *et al.* 1997, 1999), antiandrogenic activity (Carilla *et al.* 1984), antioestrogenic activity (Di Silverio *et al.* 1992), alpha-1 adrenoceptor antagonism (Goepel *et al.* 1999) and an anti-inflammatory action. However, these proposed mechanisms are not universally accepted (Rhodes *et al.* 1993; Strauch *et al.* 1994).

The placebo-controlled studies of Permixon have all been in small numbers of patients and of short duration. One study found no significant difference in LUTS, flow rates or residual urine volume between Permixon 160 mg bd for three months and placebo (Reece Smith *et al.* 1986). However, three other placebo-controlled studies of Permixon 160 mg bd found a significant improvement in urinary frequency (11–20 per cent mean reduction), nocturia (33–46 per cent mean reduction) and Q_{max} (29–50 per cent mean increase; 2.7–3.4 ml/s) compared to placebo (Champault *et al.* 1984; Cukier *et al.* 1985; Descotes *et al.* 1995).

The only significant comparative study between Permixon and other medical therapies in BPO is with finasteride. Carraro *et al.* (1996) in a randomised study of 1,098 patients over six months found a similar significant decrease in symptom score (a fall in IPSS of approximately 6), improvement in quality of life (38 and 41 per cent) and increase in Q_{max} (2.7 ml/s and 3.2 ml/s) from baseline with Permixon and finasteride respectively. A significant decrease in post-void residual (18 per cent) with finasteride only was seen. Prostate volume decreased by 18 per cent and PSA by 41 per cent in the finasteride group, compared with 6 per cent decrease in volume and 3 per cent increase in PSA with Permixon. Both drugs were well tolerated. This study has been criticised because of the lack of a placebo group.

Hypoxis rooperi

The active ingredient of the extract derived from the root of the South African star grass *Hypoxis rooperi* is thought to be β-sitosterol. Its mechanism of action is unknown. A randomised placebo-controlled study of the β-sitosterol extract Harzol in 200 men with BPO has been reported (Berges *et al.* 1995). A significant improvement in symptom score (mean 7.4 reduction in IPSS), mean Q_{max} (from 9.9 to 15.2 ml/s) and residual urine volume (from 65.8 to 30.4 ml) was seen with Harzol compared to placebo.

Pygeum africanum

Tadenum is a lipid-soluble bark extract of the *Pygeum africanum* tree used in the treatment of LUTS suggestive of BPO in Europe. Its exact mechanism of action is again uncertain. In animal studies of BOO it appears to protect detrusor function by inhibiting the activation of proteases, lipases and free radicals, thus protecting the integrity of mitochondrial membranes (Levin *et al.* 1996a, 1996b). An anti-oestrogenic effect (Mathé 1995) and an inhibitory effect on prostatic fibroblast proliferation (Yablonsky *et al.* 1997) have also been described.

Several small placebo-controlled studies of two months' duration or less have described significant improvements in urinary frequency and urine flow rate with Tadenum 50–100 mg daily (Andro & Riffaud 1995). The results of larger long-term studies are awaited.

Pollen extract

Cernilton is a pollen extract derived from many different plants growing in Southern Sweden, widely used in Europe for the treatment of LUTS suggestive of BPO. It may act by reducing prostatic urethral resistance (Takeuchi *et al.* 1981). Randomised placebo-controlled studies have shown significant improvements in symptoms with Cernilton compared to placebo (Becker & Ebeling 1988; Buck *et al.* 1990), with a significant reduction in post-void residual urine volume (Becker & Ebeling 1988) but no change in flow rates or prostatic volume (Buck *et al.* 1990). An uncontrolled comparative study of 89 patients randomised to either Cernilton or Tadenum for four months showed a greater improvement in mean flow rate and reduction in symptom score and residual volumes with Cernilton compared with Tadenum. Both preparations were well tolerated.

Plant extract combinations

Many different plant extract combinations are available, but few have been subjected to randomised placebo-controlled trials. Curbicin – a combination of pumpkin seed and saw palmetto berry – was evaluated by Carbin *et al.* (1990) in a randomised placebo-controlled trial of 53 patients over four months. Significant improvement in mean urinary frequency, flow rate and residual volume was seen with Curbicin compared to controls.

Prostagutt forte – a combination of saw palmetto berry and stinging nettle extract – has been compared to placebo (Metzker *et al.* 1996) and finasteride (Sökeland & Albrecht 1997) in randomised studies. Statistically significant improvement in symptom score, flow rate and residual volume was seen with Prostagutt forte compared to placebo, with similar improvements seen in the finasteride group.

Conclusions

The α_1-AR antagonists in common clinical use have similar efficacy and are well tolerated in most men, with little evidence to support claims of better clinical uroselectivity for any one α-blocker. They provide significant durable symptomatic improvement with modest increases in flow rates in most men, and are the first-line medical therapy for the treatment of LUTS suggestive of BPO.

Similar improvements have been found in men with symptomatic BPE (prostate volume >40 cc) with finasteride, with possible long-term reduction in the morbidity associated with BPO. No additional clinical benefit over α_1-AR-blockade alone is apparent when an α_1-AR antagonist is combined with finasteride. Phytotherapy in men with presumed BPO is well tolerated with modest short-term improvements in symptoms and flow rates. However, their mechanism of action remains largely unknown, and further large-scale studies are required to assess its long-term efficacy and place in the medical treatment of BPO.

References

Abrams P, Schafer W, Tammela TL *et al.* (1999). Improvement of pressure flow parameters with finasteride is greater in men with large prostates. Finasteride Urodynamics Study Group. *J Urol* **161**, 1513–7.

Abrams P, Schulman CC, Vaage S & The European Tamsulosin Study Group (1995). Tamsulosin, a selective α_{1c}-adrenoceptor antagonist: a randomized controlled trial in patients with benign prostatic 'obstruction' (symptomatic BPH). *Br J Urol* **76**, 325–6.

Abrams PH, Shah PJR, Stone R & Choa RG (1982). Bladder outflow obstruction treated with phenoxybenzamine. *Br J Urol* **54**, 527–30.

Abrams P, Speakman M, Stott M, Arkell D & Pocock R (1997). A dose-ranging study of the efficacy and safety of tamsulosin, the first prostate-selective α_{1A}-adrenoceptor antagonist, in patients with prostatic obstruction (symptomatic BPH). *Br J Urol* **80**, 587–96.

Albertsen PC, Pellissier JM, Lowe FC, Girman CJ & Roerhborn CG (1999). Economic analysis of finasteride: a model-based approach using data from the Proscar Long-term Efficacy and Safety Study. *Clin Ther* **21**, 1006–24.

Andersen JT, Ekman P, Wolf H *et al.* (1995). Can finasteride reverse the progress of benign prostatic hyperplasia? A two-year placebo-controlled study. *Urology* **46**, 631–7.

Andersson K-E, Lepor H & Wyllie M (1997). Prostatic α_1-adrenoceptors and uroselectivity. *Prostate* **30**, 202–15.

Andriole GL, Lieber M, Smith J *et al.* (1995). Treatment with finasteride following radical prostatectomy for prostate cancer. *Urology* **45**, 491–7.

Andriole GL, Guess HA, Epstein Jl *et al.* (1998). Treatment with finasteride preserves usefulness of prostate-specific antigen in the detection of prostate cancer: results of a randomized double-blind placebo-controlled clinical trial. PLESS Study Group. Proscar Long-term Efficacy and Safety Study. *Urology* **52**, 195–201.

Andro MC & Riffaud JP (1995). *Pygeum africanum* extract for the treatment of patients with benign prostatic hyperplasia: a review of 25 years of published experience. *Curr Ther Res* **56**, 796–817.

Ball AJ, Feneley RC & Abrams PH (1981). The natural history of untreated 'prostatism'. *Br J Urol* **53**, 613–16.

Barrack ER & Berry SJ (1987). DNA synthesis in the canine prostate: effects of androgen and estrogen treatment. *Prostate* **10**, 45–56.

Bayne CW, Donnelly F, Ross M & Habib FK (1999). Serenoa repens (Permixon): a 5 alpha-reductase type I and ll inhibitor – new evidence in a coculture model of BPH. *Prostate* **40**, 232–41.

Bayne CW, Grant ES, Chapman K & Habib FK (1997). Characterisation of a new co-culture model for BPH which expresses 5 alpha-reductase types I and II: the effects of Permixon on DHT formation. *J Urol* **157**(Suppl.4), 194 (Abstr. 755).

Becker H & Ebeling L (1988). Konservative therapie der benignen prostata-hyperplasie (BPH) mit Cernilton. *Urologe (B)* **28**, 301–6

Berges RR, Windeler J, Trampisch H, Senge TH & The β-sitosterol Study Group (1995). Randomised, placebo-controlled double blind clinical trial of beta-sitosterol in patients with benign prostatic hyperplasia. *Lancet* **345**, 1529–32.

Berry SJ, Coffey DS, Walsh PC & Ewing LL (1984). The development of human benign prostatic hyperplasia with age. *J Urol* **132**, 474–9.

Bosch RJ, Griffiths DJ, Blom JH & Schroeder FH (1989). Treatment of benign prostatic hyperplasia by androgen deprivation: effects on prostate size and urodynamic parameters. *J Urol* **141**, 68–72.

Bostwick DG, Cooner WH, Denis L *et al.* (1992). The association of benign prostatic hyperplasia and cancer of the prostate. *Cancer* **70**, 291–301.

Boyle P, Gould L & Roehrborn CG (1996). Prostate volume predicts outcome of treatment of benign prostatic hyperplasia with finasteride: meta-analysis of randomized clinical trials. *Urology* **48**, 398–405.

Brawer MK, Adams G, Epstein H & the Benign Prostatic Hyperplasia Study Group (1993). Terazosin in the treatment of benign prostatic hyperplasia. *Arch Fam Med* **2**, 929–35.

Brawer MK, Lin DW, Williford WO, Jones K & Lepor H (1999). Effect of finasteride and/or terazosin on serum PSA: results of VA Cooperative Study: 359. *Prostate* **39**, 234–9.

Bruskewitz R, Girman CJ, Fowler J *et al.* (1999). Effect of finasteride on bother and other health-related quality of life aspects associated with benign prostatic hyperplasia. PLESS Study Group. Proscar Long-term Efficacy and Safety Study. *Urology* **54**, 670–8.

Buck AC, Cox R, Rees RWM, Ebeling L & John A (1990). Treatment of outflow tract obstruction due to benign prostatic hyperplasia with the pollen extract Cernilton. *Br J Urol* **66**, 398–404.

Buzelin JM, Hebert M, Blondin P & the PRAZALF Group (1993). Alpha-blocking treatment with alfuzosin in symptomatic benign prostatic hyperplasia: comparison study with prazosin. *Br J Urol* **72**, 922–7.

Buzelin JM, Roth S, Geffriaud-Ricouard C, Delauche-Cavallier MC & the ALGEBI Study Group (1996). Efficacy and safety of sustained-release alfuzosin 5 mg in patients with benign prostatic hyperplasia. *Urology* **47**, 335–42.

Buzelin JM, Fonteyne E, Kontturi M, Witjes WPJ & Khan A, for the European Tamsulosin Study Group (1997). Comparison of tamsulosin with alfuzosin in the treatment of patients with lower urinary tract symptoms suggestive of bladder outlet obstruction (symptomatic benign prostatic hyperplasia). *Br J Urol* **80**, 597–605.

Byrnes CA, Morton AS, Liss CL *et al.* (1995). Efficacy, tolerability and effect on health-related quality of life of finasteride compared to placebo in men with symptomatic benign prostatic hyperplasia: the community-based urology study of Proscar. *Clin Ther* **17**, 956–9.

Caine M, Perlberg S & Gordon R (1975a). The treatment of benign prostatic hypertrophy with flutamide (SCH:13521): a placebo-controlled study. *J Urol* **114**, 564–8.

Caine M, Raz S & Ziegler M (1975b). Adrenergic and cholinergic receptors in the human prostatic capsule and bladder neck. *Br J Urol* **47**, 193–202.

Caine M, Pfau A & Perlberg S (1976). The use of alpha-adrenergic blockers in benign prostatic obstruction. *Br J Urol* **48**, 255–9.

Caine M, Perlberg S & Meretyk S (1978). A placebo controlled trial of the effect of phenoxy-benzamine in benign prostatic obstruction. *Br J Urol* **114**, 551–4.

Caine M, Perlberg S & Shapiro A (1981). Phenoxybenzamine for benign prostatic obstruction. *Urology* **17**, 542–6.

Carbin B-E, Larsson B & Lindahl O (1990). Treatment of benign prostatic hyperplasia with phytosterols. *Br J Urol* **66**, 639–41.

Carilla E, Briley M, Fauran F, Sultan C & Duvilliers C (1984). Binding of Permixon, a new treatment for benign prostatic hyperplasia, to the cystosolic androgen receptor in the rat prostate. *J Steroid Biochem* **20**, 521–3.

Carraro JC, Raynaud JP, Koch G *et al.* (1996). Comparison of phytotherapy (Permixon) with finasteride in the treatment of benign prostatic hyperplasia: a randomised international study of 1098 patients. *Prostate* **29**, 231–40.

Champault G, Patel JC & Bonnard A (1984). A double-blind trial of an extract of the plant *Serenoa repens* in benign prostatic hyperplasia. *Br J Clin Pharmacol* **18**, 461–2.

Chapple CR, Andersson KE, Bono VA *et al.* (1988). α-blockers clinical results. In *Proceedings of the 4th International Consultation on Benign Prostatic Hyperplasia* (ed. L Denis, K Griffiths, S Khour, ATK Cockett, J McConnell, C Chatelain, G Murphy & O Yoshida), pp. 610–32. Health Publications Ltd, Plymouth.

Chapple CR, Aubrey ML, James S *et al.* (1989). Characterisation of human prostatic adrenoceptors using pharmacology receptor binding and localisation. *Br J Urol* **63**, 487–96.

Chapple CR, Christmas TJ & Milroy EJG (1990). A twelve week placebo-controlled study of prazosin in the treatment of prostatic obstruction. *Urol Int* **45**, 47–55.

Chapple CR, Carter P, Christmas TJ *et al.* (1994a). A three month double-blind study of doxazosin as treatment for benign prostatic bladder outlet obstruction. *Br J Urol* **74**, 50–6.

Chapple CR, Couldwell CJ, Noble AJ & Chess-Williams R (1994b). The in vitro α_1 adrenoceptor mediated effects of tamsulosin on the human prostate. *Proc 23rd Congr Societé Internationale d'Urologie,* Sydney, 18–22 September, **210** (Abstr. 487).

Chapple CR, Wyndaele JJ, Nordling J, Boeminghaus F, Ypma AFGVM & Abrams P (1996). Tamsulosin, the first prostate-selective α_{1A}-adrenoceptor antagonist: a meta-analysis of two randomized placebo-controlled multicentre studies in patients with benign prostatic obstruction (symptomatic BPH). *Eur Urol* **29**, 155–67.

Chon JK, Borkowski A, Partin AW, Isaacs JT & Kyprianou N (1999). Alpha 1-adrenoceptor antagonists terazosin and doxazosin induce prostate apoptosis without affecting cell proliferation in patients with benign prostatic hyperplasia. *J Urol* **161**, 2002–8.

Chow W, Hahn D, Sandhu D, Slaney P, Henshaw R, Das G & Wells P (1990). Multicentre controlled trial of indoramin in the symptomatic relief of benign prostatic hypertrophy. *Br J Urol* **65**, 36–8.

Christensen MM, Husted SE, Wolf H *et al.* (1993). Doxazosin treatment in patients with prostatic obstruction. A double-blind placebo-controlled study. *Scand J Urol Nephrol* **27**, 39–44.

Chute CG, Panser LA, Girman CJ *et al.* (1993). The prevalence of prostatism, a population-based survey of urinary symptoms. *J Urol* **150**, 85–9.

Cockett ATK, Aso Y, Denis L *et al.* (1993). Recommendations of the International Consensus Committee. In *The 2nd international consensus on benign prostatic hyperplasia (BPH)* (ed. ATK Cockett, S Khoury, Y Aso *et al.*), pp. 553–64. SCI, Jersey, Channel Islands.

Craigen AA, Hickling JB, Saunders CR & Carpenter RG (1969). Natural history of prostatic obstruction. *J R Coll Gen Pract* **18**, 226–32

Cukier J, Ducassou J, Le Guillou M *et al.* (1985). Permixon versus placebo. Resultats d'une étude multicentrique. *Pharmacol Clin* **4**, 15–21.

Cunha GR, Donjacour AA, Cooke PS *et al.* (1987). The endocrinology and developmental biology of the prostate. *Endocr Rev* **8**, 388.

Debruyne FMJ, Jardin A, Colloi D *et al.* (1998). Sustained-release alfuzosin, finasteride and the combination of both in the treatment of benign prostatic hyperplasia. *Eur Urol* 34, 169–175.

Denis L, Pagano F, Robertson C, Nonis A, Boyle P & the Mepartricin Study Group (1997). Double-blind, randomised, placebo-controlled trial of Mepartricin in the treatment of BPH: final results after 6 months follow-up. *J Urol* **157**(Suppl.4), 136, A532.

Descotes JL, Rambeaud JJ, Deschaseaux P & Faure G (1995). Placebo-controlled evaluation of the efficacy and tolerability of Permixon in benign prostatic hyperplasia after exclusion of placebo responders. *Clin Drug Invest* **9**, 291–7.

Djavan B & Marberger M (1999). A meta-analysis on the efficacy and tolerability of alpha 1-adrenoceptor antagonists in patients with lower urinary tract symptoms suggestive of benign prostatic onstruction. *Eur Urol* **36**, 1–13.

Di Silverio F, D'Eramo G, Lubrano C *et al.* (1992). Evidence that *Serenoa repens* extract displays an antiestrogenic activity in prostatic tissue of benign prostatic hypertrophy patients. *Eur Urol* **21**, 309–14.

Di Silverio F, Sciarra A, D'Eramo G *et al.* (1996). Response to tissue androgen and epidermal growth factor concentrations to the administration of finasteride, flutamide and *Serenoa repens* in patients with BPH. *Eur Urol* **30**(Suppl.2), (Abstr.317).

Diokno AC, Brown MB, Goldstein N & Herzog AR (1992). Epidemiology of bladder emptying symptoms in elderly men. *J Urol* **148**, 1817–21.

Doll HA, Black NA, McPherson K, Flood AB, Williams GB & Smith JC (1992). Morbidity, mortality and complications following transurethral resection of the prostate for benign prostatic hypertrophy. *J Urol* **147**, 1566–73.

Elhilali MM, Ramsey EW, Barkin J *et al.* (1996). A multicentre, randomized double-blind, placebo-controlled study to evaluate the safety and efficacy of terazosin in the treatment of benign prostatic hyperplasia. *Urology* **47**, 335–42.

En LM & Tveter KJ (1993). A prospective placebo-controlled study of the antiandrogen Casodex as treatment for patients with benign prostatic hyperplasia. *J Urol* **150**, 90–4.

En LM & Tveter KJ (1994). Safety, side effects and patient acceptance of the luteinizing hormone releasing hormone agonist leuprolide in treatment of benign prostatic hyperplasia. *J Urol* **152**, 448–52.

Ezz el Din K, Kiemeney LALM, de Wildt MJAM, Rosier PFWM, Debruyne FMJ & de la Rosette JJMCH (1996). The correlation between bladder outlet obstruction and lower urinary tract symptoms as measured by the International Prostate Symptom Score. *J Urol* **156**, 1020–5.

Fawzy A, Braun K, Lewis GP, Gaffney M, Ice K & Dias N (1995). Doxazosin in the treatment of benign prostatic hyperplasia in normotensive patients: a multicentre study. *J Urol* **154**, 105–9.

Fawzy A, Hendry A, Cook E & Gonzalez F (1999). Long-term (4 year) effficacy and tolerability of doxazosin for the treatment of concurrent benign prostatic hyperplasia and hypertension. *Int J Urol* **6**, 346–54.

The Finasteride Study Group (1993). Finasteride (MK-906) in the treatment of benign prostatic hyperplasia. *Prostate* **22**, 291–9.

Ford APDW, Arredondo NF, Blue DR *et al.* (1996). N-2-(2-cyclopropylmethoxyphenoxy) ethyl-5-chloro-a, a-dimethyl-1H-indole-3-ethanamine hydrochloride), a selective α_{1A}-adrenoceptor antagonist, displays low affinity for functional α_1-adrenoceptors in human prostate: implications for adrenoceptor classification. *Mol Pharmacol* **49**, 209–15.

Forray C, Bard JA, Wetzel JM *et al.* (1994). The α_1-adrenergic receptor that mediates smooth muscle contraction in human prostate has the pharmacological properties of the cloned human α_{1c} subtype. *Mol Pharmacol* **45**, 703–8.

Fugslig S, Aagard J, Jonler M, Olesen S & Norgaard JP (1994). Survival after transurethral resection of the prostate: a 10-year follow-up. *J Urol* **151**, 637–9.

Fulton B, Wagstaff AJ & Sorkin EM (1995). Doxazosin. An update of its clinical pharmacology and therapeutic applications in hypertension and benign prostatic hyperplasia. *Drugs* **49**, 295–320.

Furuya S, Kumamoto Y, Yokoyama E, Tsukamoto T, Izumi T & Abiko Y (1982). Alpha-adrenergic activity and urethral pressure in prostatic zone in benign prostatic hypertrophy. *J Urol* **128**, 836–9.

Gabrilove JL, Levine AC, Kirschenbaum A & Droller M (1989). Effect of long-acting gonadotrophin-releasing hormone analog (leuprolide) therapy on prostatic size and symptoms in 15 men with benign prostatic hypertrophy. *J Clin Endocrin* **69**, 629–32.

Garraway WM, Collins GN & Lee RJ (1991). High prevalence of benign prostatic hypertrophy in the community. *Lancet* **338**, 469–71.

Gerber GS, Kim JH, Contreras BA, Steinberg GD & Rukstalis DB (1996). An observational urodynamic evaluation of men with lower urinary tract symptoms treated with doxazosin. *Urology* **47**, 840–4.

Gillenwater JY, Conn RL, Chrysant SG *et al.* (1995). Doxazosin for the treatment of benign prostatic hyperplasia in patients with mild to moderate essential hypertension: a double-blind, placebo-controlled, dose-response multicentre study. *J Urol* **154**, 110–15.

Gingell JC, Knünagel H, Kurth KH, Tunn UW & the Schering 90.062 Study Group (1995). Placebo-controlled double-blind study to test the efficacy of the aromatase inhibitor atamestane in patients with benign prostatic hyperplasia not requiring operation. *J Urol* **154**, 399–401.

Girman CJ, Jacobsen SJ, Rhodes T, Guess HA, Roberts RO & Lieber MM (1999). Association of health-related quality of life and benign prostatic enlargement. *Eur Urol* **35**, 277–84.

Goepel M, Hecker U, Krege S, Rubben H & Michel MC (1999). Saw Palmetto extracts potently and noncompetitively inhibit human alpha 1-adrenoceptors in vitro. *Prostate* **38**, 208–15.

Gormley GJ, Stoner E, Bruskewitz RC *et al.* (1992). The effect of finasteride in men with benign prostatic hyperplasia. *N Engl J Med* **327**, 1185–91.

Greenberg RN (1986). Overview of patient compliance with medication dosing: a literature review. *Clin Ther* **6**, 592–9

Guess HA, Heyse JF & Gormley GJ (1993). The effect of finasteride on prostate-specific antigen in men with benign prostatic hyperplasia. *Prostate* **22**, 31–37.

Hedlund H, Andersson KE & Ek A (1983). Effect of prazosin in patients with benign prostatic obstruction. *J Urol* **130**, 275–8.

Hedlund H, Andersson KE & Larsson B (1985). Alpha receptors and muscarinic receptors in the isolated human prostate. *J Urol* **134**, 1291–8.

Henderson D, Habenicht UF, Nishino Y & El Etreby MF (1987). Estrogens in benign prostatic hyperplasia: the basis for aromatase inhibitor therapy. *Steroids* **50**, 219–33.

Hieble JP, Byland DB, Clarke DE, Eikenberg DC, Langer SZ, Lefkowitz RJ, Minneman KP & Ruffolo RR Jr (1995). International Union of Pharmacology X. Recommendation of nomenclature of α_1-adrenoceptors: consensus update. *Pharmacol Rev* **47**, 267–70.

Hofner K, Claes H, De Reijke TM, Folkstad B & Speakman MJ (1999). Tamsulosin 0.4mg once daily: effect on sexual function in patients with lower urinary tract symptoms suggestive of benign prostatic obstruction. *Eur Urol* **36**, 335–41.

Hudson PB, Boake R, Trachtenberg J *et al.* (1999). Efficacy of finasteride is maintained in patients with benign prostatic hyperplasia treated for 5 years. The North American Finasteride Study Group. *Urology* **53**, 690–5.

Imperato-McGinley J, Guevro L, Gauteri T & Peterson RE (1974). Steroid 5-alpha-reductase deficiency in a man: an inherited form of pseudohermaphroditism. *Science* **186**, 1213–15.

Jacobsen SJ, Jacobsen DJ, Girman CJ *et al.* (1999). Treatment of benign prostatic hyperplasia among community dwelling men: the Olmstead County study of urinary symptoms and health status. *J Urol* **162**, 1301–6.

Jardin A, Bensadoun H, Delauche-Cavallier MC, Attali P & the BPH-ALF Group (1991). Alfuzosin for treatment of benign prostatic hypertrophy. *Lancet* **337**, 1457–61.

Jensen KM, Jorgensen JB, Mogensen P *et al.* (1986). Some clinical aspects of uroflowmetry in elderly males. A population survey. *Scand J Urol Nephrol* **20**, 93–9.

Kadow C, Feneley RC & Abrams PH (1988). Prostatectomy or conservative management in the treatment of benign prostatic hypertrophy. *Br J Urol* **61**, 432–4.

Kawabe K, Ueno A, Takimoto Y, Aso Y, Kato H & the YM617 Clinical Study Group (1990). Use of an α_1-blocker YM617, in the treatment of benign prostatic hypertrophy. *J Urol* **144**, 908–11.

Kenny BA, Miller AM, Williamson IJR, O'Connell J, Chalmers DH & Naylor AM (1996). Evaluation of the pharmacological selectivity profile of α_1 adrenoceptor antagonists at prostatic α_1 adrenoceptors: binding, functional and in vivo studies. *Br J Pharmacol* **118**, 871–8.

Kirby RS (1998). Terazosin in benign prostatic hyperplasia: effects on blood pressure in normotensive and hypertensive men. *Br J Urol Int* **82**, 373–9.

Kirby RS, Coppinger SWC, Corcoran MO, Chapple CR, Flannigan M & Milroy EJG (1987). Prazosin in the treatment of prostatic obstruction. A placebo controlled study. *Br J Urol* **60**, 136–42.

Kirby RS, Bryan J, Eardley I *et al.* (1992). Finasteride in the treatment of benign prostatic hyperplasia. A urodynamic evaluation. *Br J Urol* **70**, 65–72.

Kitada S & Kumazawa J (1987). Pharmacological characteristics of smooth muscle in benign prostatic hyperplasia and normal prostatic tissue. *J Urol* **63**, 487–96.

Langdon CG & Packard RS (1994). Doxazosin in hypertension: results of a general practice study in 4809 patients. *Br J Clin Pract* **48**, 293–8.

Lepor H (1996). Terazosin in the treatment of benign prostatic hyperplasia. In *Textbook of benign prostatic hyperplasia* (ed. R Kirby, J McConnell, J Fitzpatrick, C Roehrborn & P Boyle), pp. 279–86. ISIS Medical Media, Oxford.

Lepor H & Shapiro E (1984). Characterisation of alpha$_1$ adrenergic receptors in human benign prostatic hyperplasia. *J Urol* **132**, 1226–9.

Lepor H, Auerbach S, Puras-Baez A *et al.* (1992). A randomized, placebo-controlled multicentre study of the efficacy and safety of terazosin in the treatment of benign prostatic hyperplasia. *J Urol* **148**, 1467–74.

Lepor H & the Tamsulosin Investigator Group (1996). Long-term evaluation of tamsulosin, a prostate-selective alpha$_1$ antagonist. *J Urol* **155**(Suppl.), 585A (Abstr.1099).

Lepor H, Williford WO, Barry MJ *et al.* (1996). The efficacy of terazosin, finasteride, or both in the treatment of benign prostatic hyperplasia. *N Engl J Med* **335**, 533–9.

Lepor H, Williford WO, Barry MJ, Haakenson C & Jones K (1998). The impact of medical therapy on bother due to symptoms, quality of life and global outcome and factors predicting response. Veterans Affairs Cooperative Studies Benign Prostatic Hyperplasia Study Group. *J Urol* **160**, 1358–67.

Levin RM, Riffaud JP, Bellamy F *et al.* (1996a). Effects of Tadenum pretreatment on bladder physiology and biochemistry following partial outlet obstruction. *J Urol* **156**, 2084–8.

Levin RM, Riffaud J-P, Bellamy F *et al.* (1996b). Protective effect of Tadenum on bladder function secondary to partial outlet obstruction. *J Urol* **155**, 1466–70.

Lotti T, Mirone V, Prezioso D, Bernardi M, Rapocci MP & Ruozi P (1988). Observations on some hormone fractions in patients with BPH treated with mepartricin. *Curr Ther Res* **44**, 402–6.

Lowe FC (1994). Safety assessment of terazosin in the treatment of patients with symptomatic benign prostatic hyperplasia: a combined analysis. *Urology* **44**, 46–51.

McConnell JD, Wilson JD, George FW, Geller J, Pappas F & Stoner E (1992). Finasteride, an inhibitor of 5a-reductase, suppresses prostatic dihydrotestosterone in men with benign prostatic hyperplasia. *J Clin Endocrin Metab* **74**, 505–8.

McConnell JD, Barry MJ, Bruskewitz RC *et al.* (1994). *Benign prostatic hyperplasia: diagnosis and treatment.* Clinical practice guideline No. 8. AHCPR publication No. 94–0582. Agency for Health Care Policy and Research, Public Health Service, US Department of Health and Human Services, Rockville.

McConnell JD, Bruskewitz R, Walsh P *et al.* (1998). The effect of finasteride on the risk of acute urinary retention and the need for surgical treatment among men with benign prostatic hyperplasia. *N Engl J Med* **338**, 557–63.

McNeal JE (1978). Origin and evolution of benign prostatic hyperplasia. *Invest Urol* **15**, 340–5.

McNicholas TA, Abrams P, Tammela T, Duclos JM & Berges R, for the ESPRIT Group (1998). European pressure-flow investigation of tamsulosin in men with LUTS suggestive of benign prostatic obstruction (BPO). The ESPRIT study. *Br J Urol* **81**(Suppl.4), 21 (Abstr.54).

Malenka DJ, Roos N, Fisher ES *et al.* (1990). Further study of the increased mortality following transurethral prostatectomy, a chart-based analysis. *J Urol* **144**, 224–8.

Marshall I, Burt RP & Chapple CR (1995). Noradrenaline contractions of human prostate mediated by α_{1A}-(α_{1c}) adrenoceptor subtype. *Br J Pharmacol* **115**, 781–6.

Martin DJ, Lluel P, Guillot E, Coste A, Jammes D & Angel I (1997). Comparative alpha 1 adrenoceptor subtype selectivity and functional uroselectivity of alpha-1 adrenoceptor antagonists. *J Pharmacol Exp Ther* **282**, 228–35.

Mathé G, Hallard M, Bourut CH & Chenu E (1995). A *Pygeum africanum* extract with phyto-estrogenic action markedly reduces the volume of benign prostatic hypertrophy. *Biomed Pharmacother* **49**, 341–3.

Mebust WK, Holtgrewe HL, Cockett ATK & Peters PC (1989). Transurethral prostatectomy: immediate and postoperative complications. A co-operative study of 13 participating institutions evaluating 3,885 patients. *J Urol* **141**, 243–57.

Metzker M, Kiesser M & Hölscher U (1996). Wirksamkeit eines Sabal-Urtica-Kombinationspräparates bei der behandlung der benignen prostatahyperplasia (BPH). *Urologe (B)* **36**, 292–300.

Michel MC, Bressel HU, Mehlburger L & Coepel M (1998a). Tamsulosin: real life clinical experience in 19,365 patients. *Eur Urol* **34**(Suppl 2), 37–45.

Michel MC, Mehlburger L, Bressel HU, Schumacher H, Schafers RF & Goepel M (1998b) Tamsulosin treatment of 19,365 patients with lower urinary tract symptoms: does co-morbidity alter tolerability? *J Urol* **160**, 784–91.

Minneman KP, Han C & Hollinger S (1994). Binding of ^{3}H-tamsulosin to α_1 receptor subtypes. *Proc 23rd Congr Societé Internationale d'Urologie*, Sydney, 18–22 September, **262** (Abstr.680).

Moore E, Bracken B, Bremner W *et al.* (1995). Proscar: five-year experience. *Eur Urol* **28**, 304–9.

Moore RA (1943). Benign hypertrophy of the prostate. A morphological study. *J Urol* **50**, 680–710.

Moore RJ, Gazak JM & Wilson JD (1979). Regulation of cytoplasmic dihydrotestoterone binding in dog prostate by 17 beta-estradiol. *J Clin Invest* **63**, 351–7.

Muramatsu I, Oshita M, Ohmura T, Kigoshi S, Akino H & Okada K (1994). Pharmacological characterisation of α_1 adrenoceptor subtypes in the human prostate: functional and binding studies. *Br J Urol* **74**, 572–8.

Na YJ, Guo YL & Gu FL (1998). Clinical comparison of selective and non-selective alpha 1-adrenoceptor antagonists for bladder outlet obstruction associated with benign prostatic hyperplasia: studies on tamsulosin and terazosin in Chinese patients. The Chinese Tamsulosin Study Group. *Journal of Medicine* **29**, 289–304.

Narayan P & Tewari A (1998). A second phase lll multicentre placebo-controlled study of 2 dosages of modified release tamsulosin in patients with symptoms of benign prostatic hyperplasia. United States 93–01 Study Group. *J Urol* **160**, 1701–6.

Nasu K, Moriyama N, Kawabi K *et al.* (1996). Quantification and distribution of α_1-adrenoceptor subtype mRNAs in human prostate: comparison of benign hypertrophied tissue and non-hypertrophied tissue. *Br J Pharmacol* **119**, 797–803.

Neal DE, Ramsden PD, Sharples L, Smith A, Powell PH & Styles RA (1989). Outcome of prostatectomy. *BMJ* **299**, 762–7.

Neaton JD, Grimm RH, Prineas RJ *et al.* (1993). Treatment of mild hypertension study: final results. *JAMA* **270**, 713–24.

Nickel JC, Fradet Y, Boake RC *et al.* (1996). Efficacy and safety of finasteride therapy for benign prostatic hyperplasia: results of a 2-year randomized controlled trial (the PROSPECT Study). *Can Med Assoc J* **155**, 1251–9.

Norman RW, Coakes KE, Wright AS & Rittmaster RS (1993). Androgen metabolism in men receiving finasteride before prostatectomy. *J Urol* **150**, 1736–9.

Office of Population Censuses and Surveys (1985). *Hospital in-patient enquiry.* Series MB4 No 27. HMSO, London.

Pannek J, Marks LS, Pearson JD *et al.* (1998). Influence of finasteride on free and total serum prostate specific antigen levels in men with benign prostatic hyperplasia. *J Urol* **159**, 449–53.

Peeling WB, Abrams P, Ramsey JWA *et al.* (1992). Double-blind placebo controlled study to evaluate the pharmacodynamic effect of SK&F 105657 in patients with benign prostatic hypertrophy. *Proc 10th Congr Eur Assoc Urol* **240**, 148.

Peters CA & Walsh PC (1987). The effect of nafarelin acetate, a luteinizing-hormone-releasing hormone agonist, on benign prostatic hyperplasia. *NEJM* **317**, 599–604.

Radlmaier A, Eickenberg HU, Fletcher MS *et al.* (1996). Estrogen reduction by aromatase inhibition for benign prostatic hyperplasia: results of a double-blind, placebo-controlled, randomized clinical trial using two doses of the aromatase inhibitor atamestane. *Prostate* **29**, 199–208.

Reece Smith H, Memon A, Smart CJ & Dewbury K (1986). The value of Permixon in benign prostatic hypertrophy. *Br J Urol* **58**, 36–40.

Reynard JM, Yang Q, Donovan JL *et al.* (1998). The ICS-'BPH' study: uroflowmetry, lower urinary tract symptoms and bladder outlet obstruction. *Br J Urol* **82**, 619–23.

Rhodes L, Primka RL, Berman C *et al.* (1993). Comparison of finasteride (Proscar), a 5α-reductase inhibitor and various commercial plant extracts in *in vitro* and *in vivo* 5α-reductase inhibition. *Prostate* **22**, 43–51.

Rittmaster RS, Stoner E, Thompson DL, Nance D & Lasseter KC (1989). Effect of MK-906, a specific 5α-reductase inhibitor, on serum androgens and androgen conjugates in normal men. *J Androl* **10**, 259.

Rittmaster RS, Norman RW, Thomas LN & Rowden G (1996). Evidence for atrophy and apoptosis in the prostates of men given finasteride. *J Clin Endocrinol Metab* **81**, 814–9.

Robel P, Eychenne B, Blondeau JP, Baulieu EE & Hechter O (1985). Sex steroid receptors in normal and hyperplastic prostate. *Prostate* **6**, 255.

Roehrborn CG, Oesterling JE, Auerbach S *et al.* for the HYCAT Investigator Group (1996). The Hytrin community assessment trial study: a one-year study of terazosin versus placebo in the treatment of men with symptomatic benign prostatic hyperplasia. *Urology* **47**, 159–68.

Roos NP, Wennberg JE, Malenka DJ *et al.* (1989). Mortality and re-operation after open and transurethral resection of the prostate for benign prostatic hyperplasia. *N Engl J Med* **320**, 1120–3.

Schäfer W, Tammela TL, Barrett DM *et al.* (1999). Continued improvement in pressure-flow parameters in men receiving finasteride for 2 years. Finasteride Urodynamic Study Group. *Urology* **54**, 278–83.

Schroeder FH, Westerhof M, Bosch RJ & Kurth KH (1986). Benign prostatic hyperplasia treated by castration or the LH-RH analogue buserelin: a report on 6 cases. *Eur Urol* **12**, 318–21.

Shapiro E & Lepor H (1986). Alpha$_2$ adrenergic receptor in hyperplastic human prostate: identification and characterization using [^{3}H] rauwolscine. *J Urol* **135**, 1038–43.

Shapiro E, Mazouz B & Caine M (1981). The alpha adrenergic effect of prazosin on the human prostate. *Urological Research* **9**, 17–20.

Sökeland J & Albrecht J (1997). Kombination aus Sabal und Urticaextrakt mit Finasteride bei BPH. *Urologe (A)* **36**, 327–33.

Stone NN, Fair WR & Fishman J (1986). Oestrogen formation in human prostate tissue from patients with and without BPH. *Prostate* **9**, 311–18.

Stoner E & the Finasteride Study Group (1992). The clinical effects of a 5α-reductase inhibitor, finasteride on benign prostatic hyperplasia. *NEJM* **147**, 1298–302.

Stoner E & the Finasteride Study Group (1994a). Clinical experience of the detection of prostate cancer in patients with benign prostatic hyperplasia treated with finasteride. *J Urol* **151**, 1296–300.

Stoner E & the Finasteride Study Group (1994b). Three-year safety and efficacy data on the use of finasteride in the treatment of benign prostatic hyperplasia. *Urology* **43**, 284–94.

Strauch G, Perles P, Vergult G *et al.* (1994). Comparison of finasteride (Proscar) and *Serenoa repens* (Permixon) in the inhibition of 5-alpha reductase in healthy male volunteers. *Eur Urol* **26**, 247–52.

Takeuchi H, Yamauchi A, Ueda T & Hiraga S (1981). Quantitative evaluation on the effectiveness of Cernilton on benign prostatic hypertrophy. *Acta Urol Jap* 317–27.

Tammela TLJ & Kontturi MJ (1993). Urodynamic effects of finasteride in the treatment of bladder outlet obstruction due to benign prostatic hyperplasia. *J Urol* **149**, 342–4

Testa R, Poggessi E, Taddei C *et al.* (1994). REC 15/2739, a new α$_1$ antagonist selective for the lower urinary tract: *in vitro* studies. *Neurol Urodyn* **13**, 473–4.

Thigpen AE, Silver RI, Guileyardo JM *et al.* (1993). Tissue distribution and ontogeny of steroid 5α-reductase isoenzyme expression. *J Clin Invest* **92**, 903.

Traish AM & Wotiz HH (1987). Prostatic epidermal growth factor receptors and their regulation by androgens. *Endocrinology* **121**, 1461.

Trueman P, Hood SC, Nayak US & Mrazek MF (1999). Prevalence of lower urinary tract symptoms and self-reported diagnosed 'benign prostatic hyperplasia', and their effect on quality of life in a community-based survey of men in the UK. *Br J Urol Int* **83**, 410–15.

Tsukamoto T, Kumamoto Y, Masumori N *et al.* (1995). Prevalence of prostatism in Japanese men in a population-based study with comparison to a similar American study. *J Urol* **154**, 391–5.

Tunn UW & Schweikurt HU (1989). Aromatase inhibitors in the management of benign prostatic hyperplasia. In *New developments in biosciences 5. Prostatic hyperplasia*. Walter de Gruyter, Berlin, 139–49.

Walden PD, Gerardi C & Lepor H (1999). Localization and expression of the alpha 1A-1, alpha 1B and alpha 1D-adrenoceptors in hyperplastic and non-hyperplastic human prostate. *J Urol* **161**, 635–40.

Walsh PC & Wilson JD. (1976). The induction of prostatic hypertrophy in the dog with androstanediol. *J Clin Invest* **57**, 1093–7.

Walsh PC, Hutchins GM & Ewing LL (1983). Tissue content of dihydrotestosterone in human prostatic hyperplasia is not supranormal. *J Clin Invest* **72**, 1772–7.

Wasson JH, Reda DJ, Bruskewitz RC *et al.* (1995). A comparison of transurethral surgery with watchful waiting for moderate symptoms of benign prostatic hyperplasia. The Veterans Affairs Cooperative Study Group on Transurethral Resection of the prostate. *N Engl J Med* **332**, 75–9.

Whitfield HN, Doyle PT, Mayo ME & Poopalasingham N (1976). The effects of adrenergic blocking drugs on outflow resistance. *Br J Urol* **47**, 823–7.

Wilson JD (1980). The pathogenesis of benign prostatic hyperplasia. *Am J Med* **68**, 745.

Witjes WPJ, Rosier PFWM, Caris CTM, Debruyne FMJ & de la Rosette JJMCH (1997). Urodynamics and the clinical effects of terazosin therapy in symptomatic patients and without bladder outlet obstruction: a stratified analysis. *Urology* **49**, 197–205.

Wolfs GGMC, Knottnerus JA & Janknegt RA (1994). Prevalence and detection of micturition problems among 2,734 elderly men. *J Urol* **152**, 1467–70.

Yablonsky F, Nicolas V, Riffaud JP & Bellamy F (1997). Antiproliferative effect of *Pygeum africanum* extract on rat prostatic fibroblasts. *J Urol* **157**, 2381–7.

Yamada S, Ashizawa N, Ushijima H, Nakayama K, Hayashi E & Honda K (1987). Alpha-1 adrenoceptors in human prostate: characterization and alteration in benign prostatic hypertrophy. *J Pharmacol Exp Ther* **242**, 326–30.

Yang YJ, Lecksell K, Short K *et al.* (1999). Does long-term finasteride therapy affect the histologic features of benign prostatic tissue and prostate cancer on needle biopsy? PLESS Study Group. Proscar long-term Efficacy and Safety Study Group. *Urology* **53**, 696–700.

Chapter 6

The evidence-base for surgical intervention

Mark Emberton

Introduction

Patients, their general practitioners and their urologists should feel that in the late 1990s we know considerably more about the effects (both good and bad) of prostatectomy than we did just a decade ago. Indeed, if we look back ten years we should note that there was considerable controversy on the effectiveness, safety and appropriateness of transurethral prostatectomy (TURP), the most frequently undertaken surgical intervention for the enlarging prostate. Fortunately, over the past decade there has been considerable multidisciplinary research into this area, from which we can now benefit. The knowledge allows both patients and their doctors to balance the relative benefits and risks of the procedure and make rational decisions about whether or not to have a prostate operation. These decisions are now based on precise estimates of the likely outcomes. Onto these estimates both patients and doctors can place their own values or utilities – as each patient and each doctor will almost certainly perceive each outcome in a slightly different way. This chapter takes a close look at the key advances that have taken place during the last ten years. Each of these developments have contributed to the move away from the uncertainty of the late 1980s to the confident restraint of the late 1990s.

TURP is dangerous, is done too often and many patients are left dissatisfied

It is probably fair to say that the urological community in both the USA and Europe would have carried on performing TURP for some time at rates that were increasing year on year had Wennberg *et al.* (1988) not chosen to include TURP as one of the procedures to scrutinise. He and his colleagues were interested in small (communities) and large (countries) area variations in the number of operations being performed that were, for the most part, difficult to explain. After many studies which looked at a variety of procedures, Wennberg concluded that operations that were associated with large differences in intervention rates – the chances of the same individual undergoing a certain procedure would vary depending on where he lived – did so because there was considerable professional uncertainty about when an operation *was* and when an operation *was not* justified. Try to get two urologists to agree when a TURP should be done on a man who is not in acute or chronic retention, and you will generate some discussion and considerable disagreement.

    Because much of Wennberg's work involved analysing large routinely collected data sets, he carried out several analyses of these data that were subsequently published in prestigious journals and were widely read. The most influential of these was the paper by Roos *et al.* (1989), which compared mortality after TURP with mortality after open prostatectomy (the most common procedure before TURP was developed). What they found had an impact because it was counterintuitive to most practising urologists. Not only was TURP associated with a greater number of subsequent re-operations, but it was also associated with an increased post-operative death rate compared with the open procedure. This difference persisted after a limited adjustment for age and co-morbidity. This paper, despite its limited attempts to control for known and unknown confounding, was perhaps the one that led policy makers and funding agencies (in the USA rather than Europe) to invest considerable sums in research that would address issues of appropriateness, effectiveness and safety.

An instrument for measuring the outcome of prostatectomy

It was fortunate that these concerns about TURP arose about the same time that the outcomes movement in the USA was gaining momentum. At its heart this movement was concerned with measuring the outcomes of procedures and incorporating patients' views on the outcome when it was possible to do so (Anon 1992). So important was this trend that US government agencies made huge sums of money available so that truly multidisciplinary research teams could be assembled to research-specific disease areas. Surgical treatment of the prostate was one of these areas (Ellwood 1988).

One of the key investigators charged with the task of examining the issues of effectiveness and variations between providers was Michael Barry. He started off by reviewing the various methods that investigators had used to attribute success or failure following prostatectomy (Barry *et al.* 1993). Physiological measures such as urine flow and residual urine proved to be unreliable and bore little relation to patients' own views of the outcome of the procedure. The existing questionnaires looking at patients' urinary symptoms had not been validated at all. We knew nothing of their validity (construct, criterion and content), reliability, acceptability and responsiveness. In other words, investigators had no reliable way of assessing how effective TURP was – surprising for the second most common operation performed in elderly men. Nor could they assess the many novel methods of treating lower urinary tract symptoms that were starting to be reported: drug treatments, devices such as balloons and potential alternatives to TURP such as laser prostatectomy.

The response was the development and validation of the American Urological Association symptom score (Barry *et al.* 1992): an index score consisting of seven equally weighted questions that generated a score ranging from 0 (no symptoms) to 35 (very symptomatic). Since its first description, it has been translated into several languages and undergone cultural validation in each new setting. It has since been endorsed by the World Health Organization and has become known as the International Prostate Symptom Score (IPSS). The description, validation, promotion and subsequent universal acceptance of this method of evaluating outcome following prostatectomy represent the most important breakthrough this decade. The availability of this instrument makes it possible to evaluate this procedure in a reproducible and relevant way for the first time in history.

Just how good is TURP compared to watchful waiting?

The availability of symptom scores permitted the use of a relevant outcome measure for use in clinical trials. Most men would have an operation in order to benefit from a reduction in urinary symptoms and the bother that those symptoms caused them. Use of the IPSS meant that patients themselves would describe their symptoms before and after prostatectomy. Patients could be the arbiters of operative success or failure. This was put to quick use by the pharmaceutical industry so the efficacy of drug preparations could be assessed using patients' perceptions rather than physiological measures alone.

In order to determine just how effective TURP was compared to watchful waiting, investigators from the Veterans Affairs Department used symptoms scores combined with bother scores in an experimental design, using watchful waiting as a comparator (Wasson *et al.* 1994). This was a landmark study. It could not have been done without symptom scores (they used a prototype to the IPSS), nor would it have provided the rich information it subsequently did without the ambitious use of a randomised design. It taught us that in the group of men studied (men with moderate symptoms) watchful waiting was safe for the patient (no additional mortality) but carried a ten-times greater risk of acute urinary retention and was not associated with any reduction in urinary symptoms. TURP, on the other hand, was associated with a significant reduction in symptoms, a reduction in residual urine estimation, and protection from acute urinary retention. Moreover, those patients who reported the greatest bother associated with their urinary symptoms had the greatest benefit. This study has proven to be most useful because it allows urologists to have a detailed discussion with patients about the precise risks and benefits associated with either having or not having a TURP.

An attempt to reduce variation in practice

Once the above were in place – a reliable method of assessing outcome and some experimental studies under way – professional bodies were keen to find out what type of outcomes were being generated in the many different types of hospitals where TURP was being performed. Some of these studies looked at complications (Mebust *et al.* 1989; Thorpe *et al.* 1994), others looked at symptomatic outcome (Emberton *et al.* 1996). All these studies demonstrated what many suspected – that large variations in the pattern and possibly quality of care were evident. This resulted in an international cottage industry that published and disseminated guidelines on how to investigate and treat men with lower urinary tract symptoms suggestive of benign prostatic hyperplasia. In the USA the money was found to generate guidelines that were comprehensive, well researched and widely disseminated (McConnell *et al.* 1994). In the UK two different types of guidelines were produced. One was aimed at purchasers (NHS Centre for Reviews and Dissemination 1995), the other at urologists (Royal College of Surgeons of England 1997). The first of these was essentially a literature review that elegantly summarised the evidence in four–five pages. It was important because it raised a research agenda and highlighted how few transurethral incisions of the prostate were performed in the UK. This is expanded upon below. The second was useful to urologists because it graded the quality of the evidence on which each statement was based. In general most statements were supported by poor-quality evidence or by expert opinion. Both have helped to create standards against which audit might be carried out, though there is little published evidence that this has taken place.

How might TURP be improved?

Although (in 1999) TURP is thought by many to be the gold standard, there is considerable room for improving the procedure. We can say with confidence now, thanks to John Wasson's report of the Veterans Affairs Cooperative Study (Wasson *et al.* 1994), which randomised men to TURP or watchful waiting, that erectile dysfunction is not caused by TURP. With over 900 patient years of follow-up, rates of erectile dysfunction were distributed equally between those men who underwent TURP or had watchful waiting. TURP does not cause erectile dysfunction. It does cause sexual dysfunction in the form of retrograde ejaculation in the majority. Provided men are warned about this and have completed their families this is not usually a problem. Some men, however, will complain of orgasmic dysfunction or loss of ejaculatory sensation (Dunsmuir & Emberton 1997). Techniques that preserve the bladder neck and pre-prostatic sphincter will prevent this happening.

Some urinary incontinence, when there was none before, is a problem in a minority of men following TURP (Emberton *et al.* 1996). This is usually not a problem for the majority of men, who experience a good symptomatic outcome and when the leakage is manageable. In approximately 0.5–1 per cent of cases gross urinary leakage results which is devastating for the patient and invariably will require some form of reconstructive procedure. Procedures that are non-destructive and preserve the external sphincter completely will result in lower rates of urinary incontinence.

Excessive bleeding (5 per cent) and serious sepsis (2 per cent) are the operation-specific complications that most commonly result in a prolonged length of stay. The former was effectively reduced by using various forms of laser to coagulate or evaporate tissue. Despite numerous trials that have demonstrated this, few people are using lasers at present because they are more expensive, result in prolonged catheterisation and may result in higher long-term re-operation rates. TURP has been modified by altering the way that energy is released into the prostate. By using higher energy focused on a smaller surface area, prostate tissue can be vaporised rather than electrocauterised. This results in much less bleeding, but longer catheterisation is often required and the procedure takes a little longer to perform.

Subtle changes in the way an operation is performed often go unnoticed. These changes may also influence outcome. Discussions with senior urologists suggest that historically it was the norm to remove considerably more prostatic tissue than is currently the case. More complete resections are associated with higher rates of capsular penetration, prolonged resection times and perhaps more bleeding. On the other hand, a more complete resection may result in a reduced need for subsequent re-operation. There are numerous other minor modifications which might be called trends, because they are adopted by the majority and become incorporated over time. It is almost impossible, however, to attribute changes in outcome to these apparent trends.

In many cases a TURP is not required at all. If the prostate is small (and half of those that undergo TURP are), then a transurethral incision of the prostate may be all that is required. If this is performed, it will result in a safer, shorter and therefore less costly procedure than TURP, and in the carefully selected patient it will be just as effective (Reihmann *et al.* 1995).

The future role of TURP

TURP is not ready to be eclipsed by an alternative technology. It is undergoing evolution as improvements in optics and energy delivery systems come about. These refinements enable TURP to be carried out with greater safety, though there is considerable room for improvement. The patient undergoing TURP in the future is very likely to have failed previous strategies aimed at reducing his urinary symptoms or relieving his acute or chronic retention. Typically, he will have tried drug treatment and failed. He may have either tried or declined to have an alternative to TURP, microwave or interstitial therapy. Alternatively, he may be experiencing one of the late complications of benign prostatic hyperplasia, such as acute urinary retention or renal failure. It is likely that the patient undergoing TURP in the future will be older, probably be treated at a later stage in the natural history of the condition and possibly have additional co-morbidities compared with his historical counterparts. This increased case severity could lead to more complex cases and additional complications. Only careful case selection and further technical and anaesthetic refinement of TURP will prevent this happening.

References

Anon (1992). Outcomes and PORTs. *Lancet* **340**, 1439.

Barry M, Fowler F, O'Leary M, Bruskewitz R, Holtgrewe H, Mebust W, Cockett A *et al.* (1992). The American Urological Association's symptom index for benign prostatic hyperplasia. *J Urol* **148**, 1549–57.

Barry M, Cockett A, Holtgrewe L, McDonnell J, Sihelnik S & Winfield H (1993). Relationship of symptoms of prostatism to commonly used physiological and anatomical measures of the severity of benign prostatic hyperplasia. *J Urol* **150**, 351–8.

Dunsmuir WD & Emberton M (1997). Surgery, drugs and the male orgasm. *BMJ* **314**, 319–20.

Ellwood P (1988). A technology of patient experience. *N Engl J Med* **318**, 1549–56.

Emberton M, Neal D, Black N, Fordham M, Harrison M, McBrien M, Williams R, McPherson K & Devlin H (1996). The effect of prostatectomy on symptom reduction and quality of life. *Br J Urol* **77**, 233–47.

McConnell J, Barry M, Bruskewitz R, Bueschen A, Denton S, Holtgrewe H, Lange J, McClennan B, Mebust W, Reilly N, Roberts R, Sacks S & Wasson J (1994). *Benign prostatic hyperplasia: diagnosis and treatment.* Agency for Healthcare Policy and Research, Maryland.

Mebust W, Holtgrewe H, Cockett A & Peters P (1989). Transurethral prostatectomy: immediate and postoperative complications. A co-operative study of 13 participating institutions evaluating 3885 patients. *J Urol* **141**, 243–247.

NHS Centre for Reviews and Dissemination (1995). Benign prostatic hyperplasia *Effective Health Care Bulletin* **2**(2). NHS Centre for Reviews and Dissemination, York.

Reihmann M, Knes JM, Heisey D *et al.* (1995). Transurethral resection versus incision of the prostate: a randomised prospective study. *Urology* **45**, 768–75.

Roos N, Wennberg J, Malenka D, Fisher E, McPherson K, Anderson T, Cohen M & Ramsey E (1989). Mortality and reoperation after open and transurethral resection of the prostate for benign prostatic hypertrophy. *N Engl J Med* **320**, 1120–4.

Royal College of Surgeons of England (1997). *Guidelines on management of men with lower urinary tract symptoms suggesting bladder outflow obstruction.* Royal College of Surgeons of England & British Association of Urological Surgeons, London.

Thorpe A, Cleary R, Coles J, Vernon S, Reynolds J & Neal D (1994). Morbidity and mortality in 1400 transurethral prostatectomies carried out in the Northern Region Health Authority. *Br J Urol* **74**, 559–65.

Wasson J, Bruskewitz R, Elinson J, Finn S, Henderson W, Reda D, Keller A, Fallon B & Stepp C (1994). The Department of Veterans Affairs Cooperative Study of Transurethral Resection for Benign Prostatic Hyperplasia. A comparison of quality of life with patient reported symptoms and objective findings in men with benign prostatic hyperplasia. *J Urol* **150**, 1696–700.

Wennberg J, Mulley A, Hanley D, Timothy R, Fowler J, Ros N, Barry M, McPherson K, Greenberg E, Soule D, Bubloz T, Fisher E & Malenka D (1988). An assessment of prostatectomy for benign urinary tract obstruction: geographic variations and the evaluation of medical care outcomes *JAMA* **259**, 3027–30.

A recent abstract (McAllister *et al.* 1998) indicates that at five years' follow-up, 15 of 38 patients undergoing ELAP required further surgery compared to only six out of 32 patients who had undergone TURP.

In general the laser prostatectomy produces a significant improvement in flow rate and symptom score in the short term. Long-term failure rates currently seem to be much worse than for TURP.

Transurethral microwave therapy of the prostate (TUMT)

There are many studies reporting the short-term results of TUMT. Recently, three studies with a follow-up of more than four years post-TUMT have been published (Glass *et al.* 1998; Hallin & Berlin 1998; Lau *et al.* 1998). We will not discuss one of these further (Glass *et al.* 1998) due to various problems with interpreting its results, some of which have been highlighted in an editorial comment (Cranston 1998). The other two studies (Hallin & Berlin 1998; Lau *et al.* 1998) both had mean follow-up periods of four years or more. Improvement in symptom scores at four years was 37 per cent and 56 per cent respectively. Mean peak flow rates in one study (Hallin & Berlin 1998) fell by 1.9 ml/sec, while in the other study they increased by 3.1 ml/sec. After excluding patients who either developed other conditions, or died or were lost to follow up, treatment failure occurred in 55–63 per cent of patients at four years.

Transurethral needle ablation of the prostate (TUNA)

TUNA uses low-energy radiofrequency delivered to the prostate via small needles inserted into the prostate at cystoscopy. Initial results (Oesterling *et al.* 1997) indicate that symptom score is reduced by about 50 per cent and peak flow rate increased by 65 per cent from baseline, at one year. Treatment failure has been reported at around 14 per cent at two years (Schulman & Zlotta 1997).

Transuretheral electrovaporisation of the prostate (TUVP)

TUVP is a modification of TURP that uses a roller-ball electrode with high current to vaporise the prostate. It is now becoming used in conjunction with TURP. The results of TUVP appear to be similar to those of TURP up to one year (Hammadeh *et al.* 1998).

Discussion

The evidence presented in this chapter demonstrates that surgery for BPH is an effective treatment option, both clinically and economically. However, with the advent of drug therapy, its indications are now being widely debated.

The absolute indications for surgery in patients with BPH are refractory urinary retention, recurrent urinary tract infection, recurrent persistent gross haematuria, bladder calculi and renal insufficiency secondary to a BPH-induced obstructive uropathy (McConnell *et al.* 1994).

It is widely accepted that surgery is more effective than medical therapy in relieving the symptoms of BPH. However, many symptoms do not severely affect a patient's quality of life and so patients are happier to accept a treatment option that, although less efficacious, carries a lower risk. Thus the severity of a patient's symptoms is often the major determining factor in their choice of treatment.

With this in mind, it could be argued that improvement in symptom score is the single most important factor in assessing the success of relative treatments for BPH, and that improvement in variables such as peak flow rate is not as essential. Taking this argument to an extreme perhaps, we should prescribe drugs that alter a patient's perception of their condition rather than address the underlying problem. It would seem sensible to us that a treatment should both improve a patient's symptoms and attempt to return their micturition to as physiologically normal as possible.

Overall, it has been clearly demonstrated by several authors that surgery is clinically and economically the most efficacious treatment option in the management of BPH in the long term. Generally, it seems from the literature that 'long term' implies a life expectancy of greater than ten years. Life expectancy in the UK for all males, irrespective of health status, is currently 18.4 years at 60, 11.5 years at 70 and 6.6 years at 80 (Office for National Statistics 1998). One would expect that an otherwise fit and well 80-year-old man is likely to live longer than a peer with severe concomitant disease. We should not therefore exclude people over 80 from surgery. Indeed, a recent study by Matani *et al.* (1996) has demonstrated the safety of surgery in this older group.

The projected age structure in the UK male population over the next 30 years is shown in Table 7.3. With a predicted 47 per cent increase in the male population in their seventh decade, and a 70.8 per cent increase in the number of males in their eighth decade, the treatment of BPH in older people is a subject we will all have to face.

Table 7.3 Age structure of the projected UK male population

	Age range				
	40–49	*50–59*	*60–69*	*70–79*	*over 80*
Population (1,000) in year:					
1996	3,972	3,205	2,594	1,798	726
2006	4,594	3,838	2,856	1,850	865
2016	4,267	4,459	3,465	2,147	989
2026	3,763	4,134	4,081	2,644	1,240
Increase over next 30 years (%)	-5.3	29	57.3	47	70.8

Source: Office for National Statistics, Information & Library Service

While admiring the wealth of new, less invasive surgical treatment options, one should remember that few drugs would survive the complications of incontinence, impotence, haemorrhage, sepsis, pulmonary emboli and death, however great their economic or clinical benefits. These treatments should only be used in the setting of a clinical trial, with long-term follow-up and preferably in comparison to the surgical gold standard (i.e. transurethral resection). It is no longer acceptable for individual clinicians to try novel treatment options outside this setting. Only then can we truly be advancing the care of our patients in an evidence-based way.

Medical therapy is most certainly a welcome addition to the armamentarium of clinicians treating BPH. However, it remains relatively new, without long-term data to compare it to surgery. One of the most impressive claims of medical therapy is its ability to modify the disease process. A 57 per cent decrease in the risk of acute urinary retention in those taking finasteride for four years has been demonstrated (McConnell *et al.* 1998). This figure is calculated from an overall decrease in the risk of acute urinary retention from approximately 7 per cent (in the placebo group) to 3 per cent (in the treatment group). However, it should be remembered that between 34 and 60 per cent of patients stop taking finasteride by four years, mainly due to lack of efficacy or to side-effects.

The cost of taking 5 mg of finasteride for one year is £323.70 (British Medical Association & Royal Pharmaceutical Society 1998). Using the data from McConnell *et al.* (1998), and assuming that of the 34 per cent of patients who stop finasteride by four years in this study, one quarter stops each year, at the end of four years the drug bill for 100 patients starting in year 1 would be £112,970. Over this period 3.3 extra patients would have been prevented from going into acute urinary retention, translating to a cost of around £34,000 per patient. This figure does not take account of any other direct or indirect costs. This does not compare favourably with the total costs of prostatectomy in the UK, which has been estimated at £1,118 (Drummond *et al.* 1993) and £1,350 (Vale *et al.* 1995). This simple illustration demonstrates that although the ability of finasteride to prevent acute urinary retention is an interesting finding, alone it is not an economically viable reason to prescribe the drug.

Past experience with the introduction of TURP has shown us that as new less invasive/safer treatments are introduced, the number of patients treated increases. The majority of the economic papers quoted here suggest a massive increase in the number of patients treated with the advent of medical therapy. If in the long term medical therapy does alter the disease process rather than just delay it, this may prevent some operations. This would be especially true in those with a short (i.e. less than 5–10 years') life expectancy. However, with a failure rate of up to 60 per cent for medical therapy, this in our opinion does not look likely. We will only truly know what the best clinical and economic options are for treating BPH when much longer-term results of drug trials and the new surgical modalities become available.

In arguing our case for surgical intervention we do not propose that surgery should be performed in all cases, or earlier rather than later (because the patient will need it eventually after the medical treatments have failed, thus potentially saving the most money). Rather we hope that the option of surgery as the most effective long-term treatment can be discussed early on with the patient, when making treatment decisions.

References

Ahlstrand C, Carlsson P & Jonsson B (1996). An estimate of the life-time cost of surgical treatment of patients with benign prostatic hyperplasia in Sweden. *Scand J Urol Nephrol* **30**, 37–43.

Andersen JT, Ekman P, Wolf H *et al.* (1995). Can finasteride reverse the progress of benign prostatic hyperplasia? A two-year placebo-controlled study. The Scandinavian BPH Study Group. *Urology* **46**, 631–7.

Anson K, Nawrocki J, Buckley J *et al.* (1995). A multicenter, randomized, prospective study of endoscopic laser ablation versus transurethral resection of the prostate. *Urology* **46**, 305–10.

Baladi JF, Menon D & Otten N (1996). An economic evaluation of finasteride for treatment of benign prostatic hyperplasia. *Pharmacoeconomics* **9**, 443–54.

Bisonni RS, Lawler FH & Holtgrave DR (1993). Transurethral prostatectomy versus transurethral dilatation of the prostatic urethra for benign prostatic hyperplasia: a cost-utility analysis. *Fam Pract Res J* **13**, 25–36.

Blomqvist P, Ekbom A, Carlsson P *et al.* (1997). Benign prostatic hyperplasia in Sweden 1987 to 1994: changing patterns of treatment, changing patterns of costs. *Urology* **50**, 214–19.

Boyle P, Gould AL & Roehrborn CG (1996). Prostate volume predicts outcome of treatment of benign prostatic hyperplasia with finasteride: meta-analysis of randomized clinical trials. *Urology* **48**, 398–405.

British Medical Association & Royal Pharmaceutical Society (1998). *British National Formulary,* September.

Canadian Coordinating Office for Health Technology Assessment (1995). *Cost-effectiveness and cost-utility analyses of finasteride therapy for the treatment of benign prostatic hyperplasia.* CCOHTA, Ottawa.

Chirikos TN & Sanford E (1996). Cost consequences of surveillance, medical management or surgery for benign prostatic hyperplasia. *J Urol* **155**, 1311–16.

Cooper JW & Piepho RW (1995). Cost-effective management of benign prostatic hyperplasia. *Drug Benefit Trends* **7**, 10–33.

Cranston D (1998). Editorial comment. *Br J Urol* **81**, 382.

Drummond MF & Jefferson TO (1996). Guidelines for authors and peer reviewers of economic submissions to the *BMJ*. The *BMJ* Economic Evaluation Working Party. *BMJ* **313**, 275–83.

Drummond MF, Stoddard GL, Torrance GW, eds. (1987). *Methods for the economic evaluation of health care programmes.* Oxford University Press, Oxford.

Drummond MF, McGuire AJ, Black NA *et al.* (1993). Economic burden of treated benign prostatic hyperplasia in the United Kingdom. *Br J Urol* **71**, 290–6.

Drummond MF, O'Brien B, Stoddart GL *et al.* (1997a). Critical assessment of economic evaluation. In *Methods for the economic evaluation of health care programmes* 2nd edn (ed. MF Drummond, O'Brien GL Stoddart *et al.*), pp.27–51. Oxford Medical Publications, Oxford.

Drummond MF, Richardson WS, O'Brien BJ *et al.* (1997b). Users' guides to the medical literature. XIII. How to use an article on economic analysis of clinical practice. A. Are the results of the study valid? Evidence-Based Medicine Working Group. *JAMA* **277**, 1552–7.

Eri LM & Tveter KJ (1992). Patient recruitment to and cost of a prospective trial of medical treatment for benign prostatic hyperplasia. *Eur Urol* **22**, 9–13.

Fitzpatrick JM (1998). A critical evaluation of technological innovations in the treatment of symptomatic benign prostatic hyperplasia. *Br J Urol* **81**(Suppl. 1), 56–63

Gillon R (1994). Medical ethics: four principles plus attention to scope. *BMJ* **309**, 184–8.

Glass JM, Bdesha AS & Witherow RO (1998). Microwave thermotherapy: a long-term follow-up of 67 patients from a single centre. *Br J Urol* **81**, 377–82.

Goluboff ET & Olsson CA (1994). Urologists on a tightrope: coping with a changing economy *J Urol* **151**, 1–4.

Hallin A & Berlin T (1998). Transurethral microwave thermotherapy for benign prostatic hyperplasia: clinical outcome after 4 years. *J Urol* **159**, 459–64.

Hammadeh MY, Fowlis GA, Singh M *et al.* (1998). Transurethral electrovaporization of the prostate – a possible alternative to transurethral resection: a one-year follow-up of a prospective randomized trial. *Br J Urol* **81**, 721–5.

Hillman AL, Schwartz JS, Willian MK *et al.* (1996). The cost-effectiveness of terazosin and placebo in the treatment of moderate to severe benign prostatic hyperplasia. *Urology* **47**, 169–78.

Ilker Y, Tarcan T & Akdas A (1996). Economics of different treatment options of benign prostatic hyperplasia in Turkey. *Int Urol Nephrol* **28**, 525–8.

Jepsen JV & Bruskewitz RC (1998). Recent developments in the surgical management of benign prostatic hyperplasia. *Urology* **51**(Suppl.), 23–31.

Jepsen JV, Leverson G & Bruskewitz RC (1998). Variability in urinary flow rate and prostate volume: an investigation using the placebo arm of a drug trial. *J Urol* **160**, 1689–94.

Kaplan SA (1998). Minimally invasive alternative therapeutic options for lower urinary tract symptoms. *Urology* **51**(Suppl.), 32–7.

Keoghane SR, Lawrence KC, Gray AM *et al.* (1996). The Oxford Laser Prostate Trial: economic issues surrounding contact laser prostatectomy. *Br J Urol* **77**, 386–90.

Keoghane SR, Lawrence KC, Gray AM *et al.* (2000). A double-blind randomised controlled trial and economic evaluation of transurethral resection vs contact laser vaporisation for benign prostatic enlargement: a 3-year follow-up. *BJU Int* **85**, 74–8.

Kortt MA & Bootman JL (1996). The economics of benign prostatic hyperplasia treatment: a literature review. *Clin Ther* **18**, 1227–41.

Lanes SF, Sulsky S, Walker AM *et al.* (1996). A cost density analysis of benign prostatic hyperplasia. *Clin Ther* **18**, 993–1004.

Lau KO, Li MK & Foo KT (1998). Long-term follow-up of transurethral microwave thermotherapy. *Urology* **52**, 829–33.

Lepor H (1995). Long-term efficacy and safety of terazosin in patients with benign prostatic hyperplasia. Terazosin Research Group. *Urology* **45**, 406–13.

Lowe FC, McDaniel RL, Chmiel JJ *et al.* (1995). Economic modeling to assess the costs of treatment with finasteride, terazosin, and transurethral resection of the prostate for men with moderate to severe symptoms of benign prostatic hyperplasia. *Urology* **46**, 477–83.

Lukacs B, Grange JC, McCarthy C *et al.* (1998). Clinical uroselectivity: a 3-year follow-up in general practice. BPH Group in General Practice. *Eur Urol* **33**(Suppl. 2), 28–33.

McAllister WJ, Absolom MJ, Lawrence W *et al.* (1998). Does endoscopic laser ablation (ELAP) stand the test of time? 5-year results of a multicentre randomized study of ELAP versus TURP (Abstr.). *Br J Urol* **81**(Suppl. 4), 23.

McConnell JD, Barry MJ, Bruskewitz RC *et al.* (1994). *Benign prostatic hyperplasia: diagnosis and treatment. Clinical practice guideline.* Rockville, Maryland: US Department of Health and Human Services, Agency for Health Care Policy and Research.

McConnell JD, Bruskewitz R, Walsh P *et al.* (1998). The effect of finasteride on the risk of acute urinary retention and the need for surgical treatment among men with benign prostatic hyperplasia. Finasteride Long-Term Efficacy and Safety Study Group. *N Engl J Med* **338**, 557–63.

Marberger JM, Marshall VR, Navarrete RV *et al.* (1997). Continuous improvement with finasteride in symptomatic benign prostatic hyperplasia (Abstr.). *J Urol* **157**(Suppl.), 133A.

Matani Y, Mottrie AM, Stockle M *et al.* (1996). Transurethral prostatectomy: a long-term follow-up study of 166 patients over 80 years of age. *Eur Urol* **30**, 414–7.

Moore E, Bracken B, Bremner W *et al.* (1995). Proscar: five-year experience (published erratum appears in *Eur Urol* 1996; **29**, 234). *Eur Urol* **28**, 304–9.

Nickel JC, Fradet Y, Boake RC *et al.* (1996). Efficacy and safety of finasteride therapy for benign prostatic hyperplasia: results of a 2-year randomized controlled trial (the PROSPECT study). PROscar Safety Plus Efficacy Canadian Two year Study. *Cmaj* **155**, 1251–9.

O'Brien BJ, Heyland D, Richardson WS *et al.* (1997). Users' guides to the medical literature. XIII. How to use an article on economic analysis of clinical practice. B. What are the results and will they help me in caring for my patients? Evidence-Based Medicine Working Group (published erratum appears in *JAMA* 1997; **278**, 1064). *JAMA* **277**, 1802–6.

Oesterling JE, Issa MM, Roehrborn CG *et al.* (1997). Long-term results of a prospective randomized trial comparing TUNA to TURP for the treatment of symptomatic BPH (Abstr.). *J Urol* **157**(Suppl.), 328.

Office for National Statistics. Information & Library Service, 1 Drummond Gate, London SW1V 2QQ.

Roehrborn CG (1994). Some socio-economic issues surrounding prostatectomy: The US experience. In *Benign prostatic hyperplasia: recent progress in clinical research and practice* (ed. K Kurth & DWW Newling), pp.409–18. Wiley-Liss, New York.

Schulman CC & Zlotta AR (1997). Transuretheral needle ablation (TUNA) of the prostate: clinical experience with two years follow-up in patients with benign prostatic hyperplasia. *J Urol* **157**(Suppl.), 98.

Scott WG & Scott HM (1993). Annual cost of benign prostatic hyperplasia in New Zealand. *Pharmacoeconomics* **4**, 455–68.

Standaert B & Torfs K (1994). Economics of BPH: measuring the intangible costs. In *Benign prostatic hyperplasia: recent progress in clinical research and practice* (ed. K Kurth & DWW Newling), pp.409–18. Wiley-Liss, New York.

Vale JA, Bdesha AS & Witherow RO (1995). An analysis of the costs of alternative treatments for benign prostatic hypertrophy. *J R Soc Med* **88**, 644P–8P.

Walden M, Acosta S, Carlsson P *et al.* (1998). A cost-effectiveness analysis of transurethral resection of the prostate and transurethral microwave thermotherapy for treatment of benign prostatic hyperplasia: two-year follow-up. *Scand J Urol Nephrol* **32**, 204–10.

Weis KA, Epstein RS, Huse DM *et al.* (1993). The costs of prostatectomy for benign prostatic hyperplasia. *Prostate* **22**, 325–34.

Woodward R, Boyarsky S & Barnett H (1983). Discounting surgical benefits. Enucleation versus resection of the prostate. *J Med Syst* **7**, 481–93.

Chapter 8

Clinical and economic evaluation of competing treatment options: clinical opinion and the case for medical treatment

David Kirk

Introduction

The development of medical treatment for benign prostatic hyperplasia (BPH) has led to a complete re-evaluation of how we should manage men with lower urinary tract symptoms (LUTS) due to this condition. The role of surgery, current indications for medical treatment, its impact on management and its long-term effects all need careful evaluation. It is also necessary to consider the economics of treatment and future developments in disease management.

Transurethral resection – the gold standard?

The accepted pre-eminence of transurethral resection of the prostate (TURP) in treatment of BPH (Bishop 1994) must be questioned. TURP is a relatively aggressive intervention for a condition which is not usually life-threatening, and in one sense it replaces a pathological entity – the hyperplastic transitional zone of the prostate – with another – an iatrogenic cavity within the gland (Figure 8.1). Surgery may be the only option if there is severe obstruction. However, the end result no more recreates the 'normal' prostate than do a partial gastrectomy or vagotomy and pyloroplasty done for pyloric stenosis produce a normal stomach and duodenum.

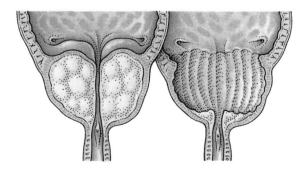

Source: Kirk D (1998). Reproduced with permission. Illustration by Philip Wilson.

Figure 8.1 TURP – schematic; hyperplastic tissue (left) removed to create abnormal cavity (right)

Although the aetiology of BPH is not fully understood, two factors are important in the production of bladder outflow obstruction: mechanical enlargement of the prostate and the functional activity of its smooth muscle (Shapiro & Lepor 1995). The medical treatments now available, albeit far from perfect, specifically address these problems – 5α-reductase inhibitors reducing the size of the prostate (Gormley *et al.* 1992) and α-adrenergic blocking drugs relaxing the smooth muscle tone (Lepor 1995). Thus, as interventions, they are more logical than is simply cutting a hole in the prostate.

The outcome of TURP

While TURP is an excellent method of relieving outflow obstruction, a substantial number of men experience problems following the operation (Roehrborn 1996) (see Table 8.1). Not only this, but there is a significant re-operation rate, reaching up to 15 per cent after eight years (Roos *et al.* 1989). Furthermore, unlike medical treatment, surgery is irreversible.

Fowler *et al.* (1988) compared the outcome of TURP in groups of men classified according to the severity of their pre-operative symptoms (Table 8.2). It should not be surprising that those who undergo the operation for mild symptoms may not find any improvement or indeed may be made worse – presumably as a result of a complication or complications of the procedure.

While TURP is the appropriate intervention for retention and for severe symptoms, for those less severely affected another approach is needed. These are the men for whom medical treatment should be considered. Although the objective changes resulting from either method of medical treatment are relatively small, they are often appreciated by the patient as an improvement in his symptoms (Holtgrewe 1998).

TURP versus medical treatment

TURP is appropriate for the most severe manifestations of the disease (e.g. refractory acute retention and chronic retention with renal failure), or where it is complicated by

Table 8.1 TURP – incidence of complications

Complication	(%)
Peri-operative mortality	0.5
Bleeding (with intervention)	2.2
Stricture/bladder neck stenosis	3.7
Retrograde ejaculation	70
Incontinence	
Stress	2.2
Total	1.0
Re-operation	>10

Table 8.2 TURP – symptomatic response depending on pre-operative symptom severity (%)

	Pre-op index			
	Acute retention	Mild	Moderate symptoms	Severe
Outcome 12-month post-op				
Mild symptoms	83	80	79	72
Moderate	11	17	15	21
Severe	6	3	6	7
Overall improvement	na	–	79	93

Source: Fowler *et al.* (1988)

bladder calculi, bladder diverticula, and recurrent infection considered due to outflow obstruction (Roehrborn 1996). Essentially, these conditions arise when the bladder outlet obstruction has caused irreversible or potentially irreversible effects on the bladder. These are manifestations of advanced disease, and our long-term aim should be to prevent them. We must, however, accept that until we have the knowledge and ability to do so, a small but significant proportion of those with BPH will present with these complications. A more relative indication for TURP as opposed to medical treatment is a severe reduction in flow rate – in the author's practice one of less than 8 ml/sec. The significance of a large residual urine (and what figure constitutes such) is less clear. Prostate size is perhaps more significantly related to disease severity than previously considered, but size *per se* is not a contraindication to medical treatment – indeed it is those with large glands who will best respond to 5α-reductase inhibitors. These issues and others are discussed by Carter in Chapter 3 of this volume. Severe symptoms are not themselves an indication for surgery; indeed, in clinical trials it is those with most severe symptoms who respond best (Gormley *et al.* 1992). However, the man with severe symptoms may well be more willing to pay the price in terms of short-term discomfort and risk of long-term complications of TURP.

Men with mild symptoms (IPSS <8) generally do not need immediate treatment. Reassurance that they do not have a serious condition and advice on fluid intake and other aspects of their lifestyle are probably enough to fulfil their needs. It is for the man with more significant symptoms but without a pressing indication for TURP, who has no inclination towards surgery, that medical treatment is indicated. The relative merits of 5α-reductase inhibitors and α-blockers are discussed in Chapter 5 of this volume. The decision will depend on whether the symptoms demand rapid resolution, the health of the patient (particularly with regard to potential interactions with α-blockers) and the size of the prostate.

Long-term outcome of treatment

Most men require treatment to relieve symptoms which are a nuisance, possibly causing a severe interference with their quality of life, but are not an immediate threat to life or health. Durability as well as efficacy is important – does medical treatment merely delay the time of the TURP? As shown in Table 8.1, TURP in no way guarantees a permanent solution. Long-term use of α-blockers has only been reported in open label studies. Although these do exaggerate the benefits, as those for whom the treatment fails will drop out, it is clear that many patients continue to benefit from α-blockers (Lepor 1995). Long-term double-blind controlled trials have been done with finasteride. The immediate effect of finasteride – the reduction in prostatic size – is measurable and has been shown to be stable over several years (McConnell *et al.* 1998). This is associated with a durable response in terms of both subjective improvements in symptom score and flow rates.

Can medical treatment reduce complications of BPH?

Many men presenting with acute retention have not sought previous advice about their lower urinary tract symptoms. Neither elective TURP nor medical treatment can have much impact on the incidence of retention in these men. However, there are data to suggest that 5α-reductase inhibitors can reduce the incidence of acute retention subsequently developing in symptomatic men (McConnell *et al.* 1998). Although there is no reason to suppose that a similar effect would not occur with long-term use of α-adrenergic blockers, and clinical trials looking at this are planned, there are as yet no data on these drugs.

The impact of medical treatment

Medical treatment is now an accepted, frequently used entity. Even in the surgically oriented urological world of the USA, it is now the first intervention used for most men with LUTS due to BPH (Holtgrewe 1998). Medicare figures have demonstrated a reduction in the numbers of TURPs done in recent years (Health Care Financing Administration 1996). This reduction has taken place despite the fact that publicity, partly engendered by the development of medical treatments, has substantially increased the number of men seeking treatment and of those with LUTS referred to urologists. In the USA, the threshold for doing a TURP has traditionally been lower than in the UK, and more men for whom medical treatment is likely to be effective will have undergone surgery. In the UK, it might be expected that medical treatment will have had less impact on TURP numbers, and certainly in Scotland, numbers of TURPs were constant for the period 1989–95 (see Table 8.3) – although this again would have been despite a rise in demand for treatment of BPH. However, even there the number of TURPs has fallen over the last two years (NHS Scottish Hospital Activity Data), providing statistical confirmation of the impression of most practising urologists that they are now doing fewer TURPs.

Table 8.3 Annual rates of TURP in Scotland

Year	No.
1989	5,919
1990	5,786
1991	5,488
1992	5,784
1993	5,820
1994	6,130
1995	5,890
1996	5,217
1997	4,173

Source: Data from Information & Statistics Division Scotland. Published with permission

Other uses of medical treatments

α-blockers are prescribed for men with retention prior to catheter removal, a use for which confirmatory clinical trial data are needed. They can relieve the symptoms of prostatodynia (de la Rossette *et al.* 1992). The less selective agents such as terazosin and doxazosin are also used to treat hypertension. Where both conditions co-exist, it has been suggested that combined treatment with a single drug is a simple and economic option (Altwein 1997). Finasteride is used as a treatment for prostatic bleeding (Puchner & Miller 1995) and, anecdotally, some surgeons prescribe it to reduce the size of the prostate before TURP, perhaps avoiding open surgery.

The risk of obscuring cancer

Does the use of non-surgical treatment run the risk of missing cases of prostate cancer? TURP does provide surgical material, which can assist in the diagnosis of carcinoma of the prostate. However, while BPH affects the central part of the prostate (McNeal 1978), cancer usually develops in the periphery and it is not uncommon to find only benign disease in a resected specimen from someone with significant cancer. Also, treatment of cancer of the prostate will often relieve associated bladder outlet obstruction, making a TURP unnecessary. Indeed, a TURP may interfere with such treatment – it will make a radical prostatectomy more difficult and complications more likely. Thus, TURP is both unreliable diagnostically and often unhelpful therapeutically in prostatic cancer.

As discussed in Chapter 4 of this volume, PSA and transrectal ultrasound-guided biopsies have largely superseded TURP, and cancer diagnosis is no longer an argument in favour of surgery. With finasteride, the reduction in PSA to 50 per cent of pre-treatment value has to be taken into account, if PSA is being monitored for any reason; however, there is no evidence that patients on finasteride are at increased risk of cancer diagnosis being overlooked (Guess *et al.* 1993). Indeed, consideration of medical treatment often encourages greater effort in excluding prostate cancer, and the generally heightened awareness of prostatic disease resulting from medical treatment has been a factor in the recent increase in carcinoma diagnosis.

Economics of BPH treatment

Surgery is associated with a substantial one-off cost, while medical treatment is continued over a number of years (see Table 8.4). Because of the relapse rate after TURP and its complications, there is a continuing average annual cost resulting from it. While it is easy to justify, on economic grounds, two years of medical treatment against the cost of a TURP, longer-term treatment will become more expensive in time. Calculations can be made to compare on a case-by-case basis the costs of different treatments. Examples are given in Table 8.4, but the overall economic argument is more complicated. Medical treatment has provided a possible therapy for those for whom previously surgery was not an option. Also, as less aggressive treatment has become available, more men with BPH are seeking treatment. Thus, while there may have been some reduction in costs from reduced numbers of TURPs, many more men are receiving treatment. It is also important to avoid escalating costs, by moving from one treatment to another – medical treatment to thermotherapy to laser prostatectomy, before the inevitable TURP. Careful assessment before starting treatment is essential, with the clear advice to the more severely affected man that one attempt at less invasive treatment, be that medical or mechanical (e.g. thermotherapy), is appropriate before a TURP.

However, there are broader aspects to the economic argument. Management of people in hospital is more expensive than in the community and the current policy of the health service is, wherever possible, to move management of patients from hospital to primary care. When surgery was the only available option for treatment, there was little incentive for a general practitioner to look after patients with BPH. The development of medical treatment has catalysed an interest in BPH in the community and should

Table 8.4 Costs of TURP versus medical treatment

	Medicare USA (1988–9)*		Economic model (2-year costs)**	
	Year 1 ($)	Year 2 ($)	Private ($)	Medicare ($)
Watchful waiting	1162	640		
Finasteride	1326	778	2,860	2,160
α-blocker	1395	845	2,422	2,161
TURP	8606	360	6,411	3,874
Open prostatectomy	12,788	69		

Sources: * Guess *et al.* (1993); ** Holtgrewe (1996)

in time lead to the majority of men with the condition being managed outside hospital (Morris *et al.* 1995). This has important implications for urological services. Urology is changing rapidly. Many other conditions are demanding the time of urologists and major surgical procedures, such as radical prostatectomy, cystectomy in the management of bladder cancer and reconstructive procedures, are increasing. Medical treatment allows patients with BPH previously managed by urologists to be taken out of the urological service, reducing the number of extra urologists needed to cope with these new demands. Here lies the true economic benefit of medical treatment for BPH.

The future

A useful analogy can be made between the management of BPH and that of peptic ulceration. Until 1975, for the latter the important effective treatments were surgical. Then the histamine H_2 antagonists (Black *et al.* 1972) were developed. Effective medical treatment was now possible, surgery declined and general practitioners became more involved in its management. With the discovery of *Helicobacter pylori* (Marshall & Warren 1984) and other developments, curative medical treatment for duodenal ulcer is now possible, with surgery retaining only a minor role.

Medical treatment of BPH is still imperfect, but as our understanding of the aetiology of the condition increases, more effective treatments will be developed and the role of surgery will gradually decline. The availability of medical treatments has heightened awareness of the condition, and is improving our understanding of the natural history of BPH. This will enable us to identify those liable to problems from advanced bladder outflow obstruction, which are the most pressing indication for TURP, at a stage before surgery is necessary. Ultimately, increased understanding of the aetiology of BPH may lead to methods by which this, the most common disease to affect men, can be prevented. Although urologists will still need to turn their hands towards TURP, and occasionally open surgery, it is quite possible that within the next 20 years the operation will be largely superseded.

Conclusions

Medical treatment of BPH is a logical approach for relieving symptoms due to bladder outlet obstruction. TURP is mainly effective in complicated BPH or with severe symptoms. It palliates rather than reversing the disease process.

TURP has a significant incidence of complications and a high re-treatment rate. Medical treatment is durable and may reduce complications of BPH.

TURP rates have fallen in the USA over the last decade and are beginning to fall in Britain too.

TURP plays little part in diagnosing cancer of the prostate.

The economics of medical treatment are complicated; increased numbers being treated may outweigh any benefits from reduction in TURP costs. However, medical treatment has catalysed community/shared urological care with an overall benefit in improving in the cost of urological services.

Future developments will improve medical management: ultimately, BPH may be preventable.

References

Altwein JE (1997). Cost-effective monotherapy of concomitant benign prostatic hyperplasia and hypertension. *Brit J Hosp Med* **58**, 592–94.

Bishop MC (1994). Are the days of transurethral resection of prostate for benign prostatic hyperplasia numbered? Alternatives still unproved. *Br Med J* **309**, 717–18.

Black JW, Duncan WA, Durant CJ *et al.* (1972). Definition and antagonism of histamine H$_2$-receptors. *Nature* **236**, 385–90.

de la Rossette JJMCH, Karthaus HFM, van Kerrebroeck PEVA *et al.* (1992). Research in 'prostatitis syndromes', the use of Alfuzosin in patients with micturition complaints of an irritative nature and confirmed urodynamic abnormalities. *Eur Urol* **22**, 222–7.

Fowler FJ, Wennberg JE, Timothy RP *et al.* (1988). Symptom status and quality of life following prostatectomy. *JAMA* **259**, 3018–22.

Gormley, CJ, Stoner, E, Bruskewitz *et al .*(1992). The effect of finasteride in men with benign prostatic hyperplasia. *N Eng J Med* **327**, 1185–91.

Guess HA, Heyse JF, Gormley CJ *et al.* (1993). Effect of finasteride on serum PSA concentration in men with benign prostatic hyperplasia: results from the North American phase III clinical trial. *Urol Clin North Amer* **20**, 627–36.

Health Care Financing Administration (1996). BESS Data. Washington, DC – cited by Holtgrewe (1996).

Holtgrewe HL (1996). Economics of benign prostatic hyperplasia. In *Textbook of benign prostatic hyperplasia* (ed. R Kirby, J McConnell, J Fitzpatrick, C Roehrborn & P Boyle), pp.527–36. Isis Medical Media, Oxford.

Holtgrewe HL (1998). The medical management of lower urinary tract symptoms and benign prostatic hyperplasia. *Urol Clin N Amer* **25**, 555–69.

Kirk D (1998). *Understanding prostate disorders.* Family Doctors Publications, Banbury.

Lepor H (1995a). Alpha blockade for the treatment of benign prostatic hyperplasia. *Urol Clin North Amer* **22**, 375–86.

Lepor H (1995b). Long-term safety and effectiveness of terazosin for the treatment of BPH. *Urology* **45**, 406–13.

Lowe FC, McDaniel RL, Chmeil JJ & Hillman AL (1995). Economic modelling to assess the costs of treatment with finasteride, terazosin, and transurethral resection of the prostate for men with moderate to severe symptoms of benign prostatic hyperplasia. *Urology* **46**, 477–83.

McConnell JD, Bruskewitz R, Walsh P *et al.*(1998). The effect of finasteride on the risk of acute urinary retention and the need for surgical treatment among men with benign prostatic hyperplasia. *N Eng J Med* **338**, 557–63.

McNeal JE (1978). Origin and evolution of benign prostatic hyperplasia. *Invest Urol* **15**, 340–5.

Marshall BJ & Warren JR (1984). Unidentified curved bacilli in the stomach of patients with gastritis and peptic ulceration. *Lancet* **i**, 1311–15.

Morris SB, Pogson C & Shearer RJ (1995). Shared care for benign prostatic hyperplasia: a feasibility study. *Brit J Urol* **76**, 77–80.

NHS Scottish Hospital Activity Data. Information and Statistics Division, Trinity Park House, Edinburgh EH5 3SQ.

Puchner PJ & Miller MI (1995). The effects of finasteride on hematuria associated with benign prostatic hyperplasia, a preliminary report. *J Urol* **154**, 1779–82.

Roehrborn CG (1996). Standard surgical interventions: TUIP/TURP/OPSU. In *Textbook of benign prostatic hyperplasia* (ed. R Kirby, J McConnell, J Fitzpatrick, C Roehrborn & P Boyle), pp. 341–78. Isis Medical Media, Oxford.

Roos NP, Wennberg JE, Malenka DJ *et al.*(1989). Mortality and reoperation after open and transurethral resection of the prostate for benign prostatic hyperplasia. *N Eng J Med* **320**, 1120–4.

Shapiro E & Lepor H (1995). Pathophysiology of clinical benign prostatic hyperplasia. *Urol Clin North Amer* **22**, 285–90.

Chapter 9

Implications of *The New NHS* White Paper for urological surgeons and general practitioners

Simon Fradd

Introduction

Aneurin Bevan defined the National Health Service (NHS) as being universally available free at the point of demand. His aspiration was that the service would lead to improved health of the general public so that the need for services would gradually diminish. In December 1997 the Labour Government published its White Paper *The New NHS*, which introduced far more radical changes than any since the inception of the NHS over 50 years ago. They are aimed at raising the standard of health care and meeting the public's aspirations. This is to be achieved through a primary care-led service. There will therefore be ramifications throughout the NHS and its associated organisations.

Historically, general practice has been funded through a separate stream from the rest of the NHS. This was written into the original 1946 Act and has continued through all its revisions. This has meant that only with the greatest difficulty could resources be moved between different heads of expenditure.

At a lower level there has been allocation of funds for revenue and capital expenditure. Most health service workers probably remember the regular rush to spend money at the end of the financial year to make sure that health authorities or trusts were not underspent.

The Conservative Government attempted to tackle this by developing fundholding. Fundholders held a single budget for the care of their patients and were able to move resources at will. (The most obvious manoeuvre was the use of savings from prescribing being used for other (supposed) patient care services.) Fundholders only controlled a small part of the total budget for their practice population. The minimum size of 4,000 patients was insufficient to allow practices to handle the potential financial risk inherent in being responsible for the funds for the total care package.

The changes

In England the development of primary care groups (PCGs) of an average of 100,000 patients is intended to overcome this problem. There will also be potential for the pooling of resources and virement between PCGs and health authorities both in year and across years. These safety mechanisms are designed to manage exceptional circumstances. PCGs will have to work within a severe financial framework and the chair of each PCG will be accountable for keeping to the allocated budget.

The New NHS Act has introduced a unified budget, with two mechanisms for moving funds from secondary services to general medical services being formalised. The first is HSG(96)31, which allows funds to be transferred from the secondary care budget (Part 1 of the NHS Act) to general practice (Part 2 of the Act) for the provision of hospital-type services in the community. A typical example is the provision of an endoscopy service in general practice.

The second is Section 36 of the Act. This again allows money to be transferred from Part 1 to Part 2, to fund the extension of primary care services. A typical example is for the management of highly dependent patients in the community, such as patients on continuous ambulatory peritoneal dialysis. The 1999 Doctors' and Dentists' Review Body report will promote several examples.

Both mechanisms are designed to reflect the change in the pattern of health care delivery and to promote further development. The Government has accepted the claims of general practitioners (GPs) that more care can be provided more effectively and cheaply in primary care. Fundamental to *The New NHS* is the role of lay and non-medical members of PCGs in determining priorities.

Drug budgets

Historically, GPs' prescribing costs have always been open-ended. Of recent times, GPs have been given an indicative drug budget. Expenditure is met directly from NHS resources and overspends taken from the Government's contingency fund outside the Part 2 allocation to primary care. Participation in fundholding was only allowed if the practice accepted a fixed drug budget.

The quid pro quo of holding a fixed budget is the ability to vire money in and out of this pool to and from other heads of expenditure. Thus lower spending on prescribing could be used to employ more staff or spend more on hospital referrals. This ability to vire funds has had some radical effects on the nature of patient care. For instance, the development of counselling services in primary care stemmed from this system.

Structure of PCGs

PCGs will have boards of up to 13 members. GPs have the right to have a majority and to hold the chair. The board will also include a chief executive, who is an employee of the health authority, another health authority member, an independent lay member, two nurses and a member from the social services department.

If no more than four GPs can be recruited, the residual places will be filled by others. There is therefore significant pressure on GPs to participate.

Initially, there are to be two levels of PCG: level 1 will be an advisory panel to the health authority; level 2 will be directly involved in commissioning secondary care. Both will be subcommittees of the health authority, but at level 2 the PCG chair will be the accountable officer for finance.

From April 2000, PCGs will be able to become trusts, known as levels 3 and 4. These will be free-standing bodies rather than subcommittees of the health authority.

At level 3 they will be responsible for all patient care, except community care. At level 4 they will be responsible for health and community care trusts.

Function of PCGs

PCGs will be responsible for commissioning primary and secondary care, for quality control under clinical governance and, at level 2, for managing their budget. The whole will be done within the framework of the *health improvement programme.*

The health improvement programme

The internal market introduced in 1990 is to be abolished. In its place will be three-year rolling programmes to improve and deliver services. This will be laid down in the health improvement programme (HImP), which will be developed by the health authority in discussion with local hospital trusts and PCGs. However, the HImP is owned by the health authority.

Each year trusts and PCGs will have to produce a report laying out their progress in relation to the HImP. They will be accountable to the health authority.

The HImP is not totally at local discretion. It must be founded on the priorities laid down in the *Health of the Nation* targets. The effect of this is that, not only will PCGs in a single health authority be working within a very similar framework, but also the difference across the country in available services and quality standards will be restricted.

Commissioning

Previously GPs have been independent contractors subject only to their terms of service and accountable to the General Medical Council. In future, general medical services (GMS) will be commissioned by the PCG. This will determine not only what services are to be provided but at what cost and to what quality standard.

Some protections have been built in. The budget for GMS is protected at the level of the health authority for capital expenditure and at the level of the PCG for revenue. However, this does not protect individual GPs or practices, although any reduction of funding is only possible after giving one year's notice.

The model for commissioning secondary care is much as it was under fundholding and commissioning pilots. The difference is that the PCG will be responsible for all secondary care, including emergencies.

Clinical governance

This is a new term to define quality of services. On the one hand, it embraces the responsibility that all health and social care providers work to a minimum standard and on the other that there is a constant effort to improve standards overall. This will be written into commissioning agreements. Previously, trusts have only had a duty to work within their budget. The duty to perform to a set standard is new.

Each PCG must have a member who is responsible for clinical governance. Their prime task will be to monitor primary care performance and assist GP colleagues to improve it. Hospitals and community trusts will be responsible for clinical governance within their organisations but accountable to the PCGs and health authority. Clinical governance will be overseen by the Commission for Health Improvement (CHI). This body will have the power to remove the boards of a trust or health authority.

Financial management

The budget is held by the health authority whose chief executive will be the responsible officer. At level 2 accountability for financial management is devolved to the PCG chair.

Funds will be allocated to PCGs under a new needs-based formula. This is to reflect the needs of local communities rather than historic spending. In the past such a formula only applied to secondary care and even then many authorities were significantly underfunded. The move to resource primary care on a similar basis is new and will be introduced gradually. The medical profession has been promised it will be done on a levelling-up basis.

Other than the increase in NHS funds announced in the Government Spending Review in 1998, there is to be no additional money for patient care or the introduction of the new management structure.

A particular concern to GPs is that the administrative work of PCGs will be far greater than for fundholding and yet this has to be completed for approximately half the cost. The Government has publicly committed itself to management savings of £200 million per year in the NHS.

The effects

These changes are undoubtedly far more than just window dressing. Fundholding was voluntary and generally involved less than 25 per cent of the total budget. The new system is mandatory and involves 100 per cent of the health care budget.

Even though significant protection of GPs' incomes has been achieved, the fact that this is at a level above the individual practice does leave GPs exposed if they do not make the system work. No other groups of health care workers have a personal investment in the infrastructure of the NHS. The average GP has £100,000 invested in premises, equipment and working capital. Already many doctors are finding the traditional model of general practice an unattractive option. Unfortunately, alternatives such as being an employee in a primary care pilot have had little uptake. There are grave concerns that the new system will make GPs feel more insecure and even more reluctant to make the necessary investment in their practices.

Unified budgets

The term unified budgets was a central feature of the White Paper. The mechanisms allow funding at PCG level to be treated as a single entity. Responsibility for working within the overall sum will rest on each and every GP. This will have vital ramifications on the secondary sector.

Prescribing costs are the most difficult item to control. Though fundholders have often made significant savings in this area, they now find they have pared spending back to the bone. Each year there are new upward pressures. New drugs such as Viagra (sildenafil) and beta-interferon are one cause. As significant are developments in clinical management. Currently, the need for the widespread use of lipid-lowering drugs is a cause for major concern.

The main pressure point is repeat prescribing. At the higher-cost end of the market this is often initiated by the hospital. The pharmaceutical industry has exploited this factor by agreeing special deals with hospital trusts, in the knowledge that ongoing prescribing will emanate from primary care at full price.

It is obvious that there will be early pressure for formularies across both hospitals and primary care. GPs who fail to live within their prescribing budget will first be advised and pressured by the PCG to come into line. If they fail to do so, the PCG has the ability to reduce reimbursement of expenses, such as rent, staff and IT costs, which are all discretionary.

Some power will have to be given to GPs to enable them to protect themselves from consultant colleagues forcing prescribing costs up. I anticipate future commissioning agreements of secondary care will link community prescribing costs with the funds available for referrals. This will have a direct effect on management protocols.

The impact of *The New NHS* on the management of LUTS and BPD

In general, the long-term trend will be the reduction in the percentage spend on hospital services. The new system is designed to encourage more care to be delivered nearer to the patient's home, of which there are already widespread examples. For instance, the radical shift of anticoagulant monitoring into the community has shown that such care is more convenient to the patient, delivered to at least the same standard and at much reduced cost. In Nottingham, during the first year of operation, over £60,000 was saved in transport costs alone and there was a considerable reduction in the amount of time previously spent by the public in travelling and waiting for transport.

The downside is that the funds for this work transfer come from the secondary sector budget. This can be accommodated where health authorities are seeing their allocations increase by more than medical inflation year on year. Unfortunately, such authorities are few and far between. In general, money has to be made available by efficiency savings or cutting back hospital services.

In urology many services can be widely transferred to GPs. Open-access laboratory services, such as flow rates and ultrasonic estimation of residual volumes, allow the GP to decide whether to manage the patient pharmacologically or by referral for surgery. This sort of change holds no great threat to the viability of urology departments. The shift in resources is small and staff losses can be dealt with through natural wastage.

Although there are already several centres with a shared care protocol, most have not yet transferred the resources that must follow this change in work pattern. Some centres may have a rude awakening.

Medical versus surgical management of BPD and LUTS

A more difficult problem is presented by the choice of treatment for urinary outflow problems. Although there are large numbers of men where the treatment of choice is medical, many still require specialist urological referral.

Considering that the cost of transurethral resection of the prostate is approximately six times the annual cost of drug therapy, in a younger patient the surgical option is by far more cost-effective in the long term than medical management. The difficulty is that health authorities are funded on an annual basis with severe limitations on their ability to raise finance against future spending.

The management of BPD and LUTS is well ahead of many other clinical conditions in the development of pharmaceutical tools. Extrapolating the arguments above to areas such as angina and more especially preventive care, there will always be pressure to deal with the here and now on a 'sticking plaster' basis rather than to deliver the most desirable clinical service.

Conclusions

There has to be a switch in Government thinking with respect to the NHS, if it is ever to deliver Aneurin Bevan's dream of such efficacy and efficiency that the service becomes largely redundant. Long-term, rather than short-term solutions must be pursued and funded. The example *par excellence* is the winter crisis funding. The NHS must have sufficient resources at its disposal to meet such foreseeable peaks in demand and use these enhanced abilities through the rest of the year to deliver a faster service which is more sensitive to the needs of individual patients.

Reading list

White Papers
The New NHS – Modern, Dependable
Our Healthier Nation
Putting Patients First
Designed to Care: renewing the NHS in Scotland
Fit for the Future

Health Service Circulars
HSC 1998/019 Practice Fund Management Allowance 1998/9
HSC 1998/021 Better Health Better Care
HSC 1998/050 National Health Service (Fundholding Practices) Regulations 1998
HSC 1998/065 Establishing Primary Care Groups
HSC 1998/120 Setting Health Authority and Primary Care Group Baselines
HSC 1998/139 Developing Primary Care Groups
HSC 1998/170 Cash Allocations for Prescribing
HSC 1998/171 The New NHS Modern and Dependable: Guidance on Health Authority and Primary Care Group Allocations
HSC 1998/179 Primary Care Groups: Clearing House Facilities
HSC 1998/190 PCG Remuneration
HSC 1998/192 Commissioning in the New NHS: Commissioning Services 1999/2000
HSC 1998/228 Delivering the Agenda
HSC 1998/230 The New NHS Modern Dependable: Governing Arrangements for Primary Care Groups

All available from health authorities and The Stationery Office, The Publications Centre, PO Box 276, London SW8 5DT. Tel: 0171 873 9090; Fax: 0171 873 8200

Department of Health website: http://www.open.gov.uk/doh/coinh/htm

GPC's PCG helpline: 0845 303 3221
e-mail: pcghelp@bma.org.uk

Index